BIRTH TRADITIONS
& MODERN PREGNANCY CARE

Jacqueline Vincent Priya has a doctorate in sociology from the University of Surrey. She has worked as a nurse, radiographer and teacher, and for fifteen years in various market research companies. During the four years that she spent in Malaysia she took the opportunity to change direction and carry out research on traditional midwifery, a subject that was very close to her heart. As a result she wrote *Birth Without Doctors* which was published by Earthscan in 1991. During her time in Malaysia she was a regular contributor to the Singaporean magazine *Motherhood* and to various Malaysian magazines and newspapers including *Medical Management* and *New Straits Times*. She is now living in Malawi with Peter and their two daughters Emma and Rachael. As well as her research and writing she is setting up and running The Birth Traditions Survival Bank.

BIRTH TRADITIONS
&
MODERN PREGNANCY
CARE

Jacqueline Vincent Priya

Foreword by
Dr Michel Odent

ELEMENT
Shaftesbury, Dorset ● Rockport, Massachusetts

© Jacqueline Vincent Priya 1992

Published in Great Britain in 1992 by
Element Books Limited
Longmead, Shaftesbury, Dorset

Published in the USA in 1992 by
Element, Inc.
42 Broadway, Rockport, MA 01966

Cover illustration courtesy the Susan Griggs Agency
Front right © Alain Evrard
Front centre © Sandra Lousada
Front left © John Bulmer
Back © Robert Frerck

Cover design by Max Fairbrother
Designed by Roger Lightfoot
Typeset by Intype, London
Printed and bound in Great Britain by
Dotesios Ltd, Trowbridge, Wiltshire

British Library Cataloguing in Publication Data
available

Library of Congress Cataloging-in-Publication Data
Priya, Jacqueline Vincent,
Birth traditions & modern pregnancy care
Jacqueline Vincent Priya.
Includes bibliographical references and index.
1. Midwives—Cross-cultural studies.   2. Childbirth—Cross-
cultural studies   3. Birth customs—Cross-cultural studies.
I. Title.   II. Title: Birth traditions and modern pregnancy care.
RG950.P75 1992   618.2–dc20   92–3038

ISBN 1–85230–321–2

CONTENTS

•

To Rachael

Who was born just as this book was
conceived, and who has grown with it
ever since.

FOREWORD

•

Watch the stars in the sky – even as you see them, some of them are already dead. Watch a documentary about the tropical forests – some species have already disappeared forever by the time they can be seen on your TV screen.

When reading this book about birth traditions you will be in the same sort of situation.

We should be grateful to Jacqueline Vincent Priya for realizing the urgency of collecting and bringing together so many beliefs, rituals and behaviours which will not survive the end of this century. Thanks to her own deep knowledge of traditional birth attendants in Thailand, Indonesia and Malaysia she has been able to compile a much-needed anthology of the most significant data collected by herself and others from all over the world.

The importance of Jacqueline's book is not purely academic. There are two reasons why it represents much more than a precious reference source for the scholars who will need it in the future. First, Jacqueline has found an elegant and effective way of combining her unique knowledge of birth traditions and her own experience as a mother to look critically at modern obstetrics. The other reason is the date of publication. This book will appear at the very time when obstetrics is in a critical phase and is seeking inspiration. By becoming scientific and, in particular, by learning to use statistics, western obstetrics is discovering its mistakes and even its fundamental weaknesses.

For the very first time we now have at our disposal scientific ways to demonstrate the importance of the effects of the environment on the period surrounding birth. Indirectly, these could enable us to rediscover the value of some traditional beliefs and attitudes. For example, we can now compare statistics from different countries and conclude that the western countries in which midwives are numerous and well-established have the best possible outcomes with the lowest rates of caesarean section. In other words, it is now possible to demonstrate in a scientific way something that has been recognized throughout the ages – that there is a world of difference between a female and a male environment in the period surrounding birth.

At the same time, many studies confirm statistically that the only effect of electronic foetal monitoring is to increase the incidence of caesarean section. In other words, an electronic environment makes birth more dangerous so that it becomes necessary to rescue more babies. There is no excuse now to advise women to give birth surrounded by electronic machines.

We are embarking upon an important period in the history of childbirth when the main task will be to prepare for the post-electronic age. Let us add that several medical disciplines outside obstetrics, especially in the fields of cancer and drug addiction, are beginning to suspect that there may be long-term ill-effects from the drugs administered during labour.

It is in this context of crisis, at a time when new priorities have to be clearly defined, that *Birth Traditions & Modern Pregnancy Care* is published. Of course, no-one would argue that we should copy the rituals, beliefs and practices of this or that culture; nor should it be suggested that we should reintroduce the strategies most known cultures have devised to deny the mammalian need for privacy in the period surrounding birth (e.g. through the belief that colostrum is harmful, etc.). Nobody in our society is about to believe that walking under the belly of a camel can help a woman to have an easy delivery. Our belief systems are specific to our own society. Our family structures have no model in other cultures. And we are able to fall back on a safe technique for caesarean section, which is the main advance in the field of childbirth during the twentieth century.

But during the same period there has been no improvement at all in our understanding of the physiological processes of birth. This is the task of the day. To do so we have to pose questions which are absolutely new for medically trained birth attendants in the industrialized countries. Is there a particular sort of food which can make birth easier or more difficult? This is an example of a basic question that might arise in a culture other than ours, but it is a new one for modern medical research. How should we select women who wish to become midwives? According to their academic background? According to their experience as mothers?

Jacqueline's mission is not to suggest any useful model which might emerge from the enormous amount of data she has collected here. Her aim is primarily to stimulate our curiosity. And curiosity leads to questions. This book will work as a catalyst. We need to provoke the right questions at the right time. The answers will follow.

Michel Odent

INTRODUCTION

•

I first became interested in traditional midwives and their work in 1986 when I went to live in Malaysia with my partner Peter and daughter Emma who was then one year old. As a result of reading various articles about them in the local Malaysian papers I thought it would be interesting to meet one. I asked a local friend to take me to see Buleh, a local practitioner from a traditional Malay village close to Seremban where we were living. This meeting affected me profoundly and as a result I decided to widen my explorations and embarked on research which led to me meeting with and talking to traditional midwives in various ethnic groups from Thailand, Indonesia and of course Malaysia. After two years I wrote *Birth Without Doctors – Conversations With Traditional Midwives* which was published by Earthscan in February 1991.

In talking with these traditional practitioners, I was always interested to see if they had any practices or any knowledge which would be of interest or use to women giving birth in the west. This had a particularly personal interest for me when I became pregnant for the third time during my last fieldwork trip in Indonesia! To explore this subject in more detail I started to look at other research which had been carried out on traditional midwives in other parts of the world and to find out more about birth traditions generally. At the same time I also started examining the history of our own system of medical care; its philosophic basis, the history of its growth, its social and psychological consequences both for individual women and society as a whole. At first it seemed that there was little in common between traditional beliefs and modern obstetrics, but as I looked more deeply into the subject, connections became evident and it is from these that the theme of this book developed.

The material for this book thus comes from several sources, the first being my own research with traditional midwives in south-east Asia. It was this that alerted me to the richness of their traditions and practices as well as inspiring me to look at the subject from a wider perspective. As a result I have sought out a very wide range of other material ranging from academic research reports to impressions from travellers of various kinds making contact with traditional groups for the first time. I have also included historical data about European and American traditions although often this was written up under the heading of 'folklore'. It was, of course, impossible to be comprehensive, but I have attempted to obtain material from as wide a range of different cultures and traditional groups as possible. I have also included research on modern obstetrics which incorporates information about its growth and history as well as scientific studies on the efficacy of various obstetric procedures.

In looking at the data from traditional societies I was frequently struck by the fact that it was gathered by men, usually as a sideline to some other line of enquiry. This was particularly true of much of the first anthropological research which was carried out mainly by men and tended to focus on masculine aspects of the society. As birth in traditional societies is usually the concern of women with men having only a peripheral role, I felt that the validity of some of this data must be open to question. In some cases it was given to the researcher by other men so it is not as full or as detailed as if it had come directly from women, and where women talked directly to a male researcher it is difficult to know the extent to which this had inhibited their responses. Fortunately there are increasing numbers of female anthropologists and social researchers who are interested in and have carried out research with women in these societies, in some cases revisiting groups which had only been looked at by men. Wherever possible I have used their work but in some cases the original data collected by men is all we have.

Throughout this book I have talked about 'traditional societies' in contrast to 'the west' or 'industrial societies'. The former I take to be people who live in small groups, usually based on family ties. They grow most of their own food and satisfy most of their needs from their own intellectual and material resources. The latter I take to be the societies as found in the UK, America or Australia where people live in large urban areas, usually in small nuclear families and who satisfy their material needs by going out to work and spending the money earned on food and goods produced by industrial processes. This is a somewhat simplistic definition as most countries now manifest both kinds of society with urban areas appearing more industrial and 'modern' and groups living in the country appearing more 'traditional'. Also, of course, traditional societies are not untouched by modern developments and all of the villages I visited had been modified in some way by the twentieth century, although often their traditional beliefs remained surprisingly robust.

Most of the research that I describe was carried out by a researcher in a small group at a particular time. Although for convenience I sometimes write that 'Gypsy women believe . . .' it does not necessarily follow that all gypsy women have the beliefs described. There are differences between individuals and groups in traditional societies just as there are similar differences in western societies. I have also tended to talk about groups in the present tense unless the data I am using is obviously historical. This is not to imply, however, that the traditions I describe are continuing unchanged or that a majority of people in those societies necessarily subscribe to them. Modern ideas and in particular those of biomedical medicine are changing them as it changed us in the west. One of the strongest reasons for my continuing interest and research on the subject of birth traditions is the need as I see it to document what is a rich heritage of female traditions before they are swept away by the forces of 'progress' and 'development' and disappear completely.

There are many people who have helped me with the research and writing of this book. In particular, I should like to thank Dang who helped me with the interviewing in Thailand, and Letchumi who helped me with interviewing in Indonesia and Malaysia. Both of them made wonderful travelling companions and became good friends. As I live abroad my access to library material is somewhat limited and I have had to depend greatly on Amanda Croome to find the articles and books that I needed from libraries in England. As I wrote this book I was continually impressed by the efficient and thorough way in which she had collected the data. I continued to be grateful for her businesslike way in dealing with all my queries at long distance and I am especially thankful for all the help she provided.

This book was written while I was living in the Yemen against a background of considerable uncertainty because of Saddam Hussein's excursion into Kuwait. I finished writing two days before we were flown back to England just prior to the start of the Gulf War. I am extremely grateful for the support I received from my partner Peter and daughters Emma and Rachael which enabled me to do this. Finally, I have a very special thanks to the midwives who shared themselves and their knowledge so generously with me and from whom the inspiration came to write this book.

Jacky Vincent Priya

CHAPTER ONE

WHERE DO BABIES COME FROM?

•

Birth, like death, is universal, but the way that it is experienced, interpreted and explained is not. The physical process is similar for everyone, but an individual's experience, how a woman interprets the meaning of the events for herself and explains what is happening within her, varies widely.

When I first became pregnant, like most of my friends who had been born and brought up in England, I focused primarily on what was happening to me physically. As my body softened and bulged I avidly read all the books I could find about the subject. These explained in great detail the physical facts of conception, pregnancy and birth, the problems I might experience and how they would be managed by the medical profession. Psychological, emotional and social factors were also discussed, of course, but like the books, I saw these as separate from and subsidiary to the physical event. With a new life growing inside me and especially in the days immediately after giving birth, I did have some strong spiritual feelings, but these were very fleeting and seemed very remote from what was happening in my body. This view of my reality was, of course, reinforced by the medical care I received which focused on the physical process of safety extracting a healthy baby. Little attention was paid to me as a person, for childbirth was seen as primarily a physical event in which psychological, emotional, social and spiritual

factors were entirely separate and only of peripheral importance.

Many years later, when I began talking to women from
traditional societies, I came to understand and appreciate a
different reality about childbirth which was diametrically
opposed to my own. Giving birth was, for them, an experience in which no distinction was made between the physical,
psychological, social or spiritual; where each aspect was
viewed as equally necessary and equally valid. The physical
acts of conception, pregnancy and birth were but one aspect
of a cycle in which social, individual and divine forces all
played a part. This cycle mirrored the cycle of birth, growth
and death which they saw in the natural world around them
and derived from their traditional wisdom about the nature
of life and death. For these women to give birth was to
participate in the mystery of life on earth and this was recognized not only by themselves but by the people who helped
them give birth, as well as the rest of the people in the
community in which they lived.

In most but not all traditional cultures, sexual intercourse
is understood to be the first step towards conception, but is
usually on its own thought to be insufficient to bring about
the creation of a new human being. For this, other divine
forces are seen to be necessary. Talking to Muslim Palestinian
women in the 1940s, Granquist[1] was told how Allah and the
angels are involved. Man is created from dust and only if
God allows can this be infused with the spark of life. As one
woman put it, 'The man sleeps with the woman but only
God can create . . . it is God who feeds her with sons'. Prior
to conception the angels bring dust from three places; the
place of creation, the place where the person will be born
and the place where she will eventually die, all of which is
decided by Allah. At conception the angel brings this dust,
kneads it and puts it into the woman's body during sexual
intercourse and it is from this that the individual develops.
After birth a person wanders in different parts of the world
but as the time for death draws near she will be drawn to
that part of the earth from which the dust for her original
conception was taken. When a person dies a long way from

home it is because this is the place from which the original dust for her creation was obtained and it is there she must return to die.

Given the spiritual forces which are at work around the point of conception it is very important that both the man and woman are spiritually pure at this time. To ensure that this is so, God's name should be called upon during sexual intercourse so that 'the devil will be made small' and will not adversely interfere with the conceptual process. If this is not done the child may be born 'with the devil in him' which could have a disastrous effect on his life as there is nothing he can do to neutralize such strong negative forces.

The Karen (one of the hill tribes in northern Thailand) also believe that one's life and the nature of one's death is decided before birth. Before being born the child's spirit decides how long she is going to live and how she is going to die. Whatever an individual's death is like it was the person's own choice about how, when and where it was to occur. There is, therefore, no need to lament a death which seems to have come too soon or was violent as it was the person herself who chose it.

Amongst the Dinka, a tribe in the Sudan, a new life is created by much more than just the mother and father. Conception is the outcome of the combined activity of God, the ancestors and the man, all of which takes place inside the woman's body. A child belongs to the lineage; to a long line which involves all the deities, the ancestors and those still to be born. It is not for the couple alone to decide whether or not to have children as this is the prerogative of God and the ancestors. The latter are thought to be the most important as they have the most interest in ensuring that the family tree flourishes by bringing more children into the world.

In other places it is the spirit of the child which plays a more active role. In Thailand, successful conception will not take place unless the soul (khwan) of an unborn human flies into the body of a woman during sexual intercourse and lodges itself in the womb at the moment of conception. The soul will be that of someone who has lived many times before, in the process of which she will have acquired an

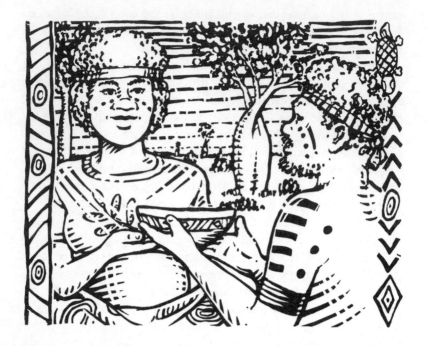

amount of merit or sin according to her actions in previous lifetimes. The fact that she desires rebirth, however, is evidence that she has insufficient merit to reach the highest disembodied planes of existence and so seeks another physical life to achieve this end. The new life as a human provides her with a fresh start but her character and heart will already have been formed from previous existences. At the time of conception, the pregnant woman may have a strange dream which is a token showing whether the child will be a boy or a girl with good or bad characteristics and what sort of person he or she will grow up to be.

In some societies sexual intercourse is considered to be irrelevant to the process of conception. Amongst the Australian aborigines, for example, the spirits of the children to be born are taken in through the food. Here, human children are the physical embodiment of the spirit children (*djnganaracny*) who were placed in the pools by the rainbow serpent in the Time Long Past before there were people. Prior to being born as a human being the spirit may have been temporarily incarnated as an animal, bird, fish or reptile. When the child is born as a human her body may have a birthmark, mole or dimple which will be the scar of the wounds that she received from the spears of men in previous incarnations. Each lineage or group of families is associated with an animal, bird, fish or reptile and both the incarnations and the lineage into which the child will eventually be born as a human will be associated with the same living thing.

As spirit children, they wander and play all over the country; some say they look like little children the size of a walnut while others say they resemble small red frogs. Conception occurs when one enters a woman through the food which is given to her by her husband. The presence of the spirit child in the food makes her vomit and later she or her husband may dream of the spirit child and maybe also the animal or reptile to which it is connected. Later, the food in which the spirit child was passed to her or the animal or reptile connected to the child will become the child's conception totem and an important part of the child's spiritual life. The man who provides the food in which the spirit child is passed to the woman is considered to be the spiritual father of the child. Although the sexual intercourse that he has had with his wife has prepared the way for the spirit child to lodge within her body, this is the only connection that it has with the conception. It is the constant proximity of the man to the woman during the pregnancy which moulds the child's physical features so that they are similar to the father's.

The Trobriands are a small group of islands in the Pacific Ocean and the explanation which these islanders have of where babies come from is a wonderful fusion of the spiritual, environmental, social and physical which makes sense of every aspect of giving birth.

When a Trobriand Islander dies she goes to the island of the dead called Tuma. Here she leads the same sort of life as she did on earth, but much happier. She ages and becomes old and feeble but by bathing in sea water the wrinkled skin of old age is sloughed off, she becomes young again and life can continue as before.

When a spirit becomes tired of constant rejuvenation,

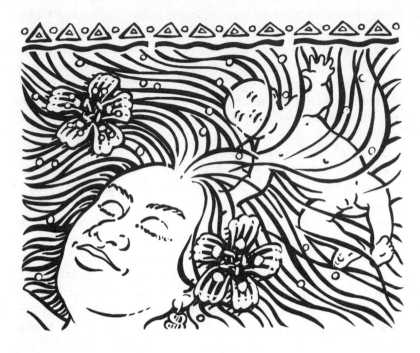

when she has had a long existence 'underneath' as the people
call it, she may want to return to earth again. When this
happens she leaps back in age and becomes a small preborn
infant called *waiwaia* which means 'infant' or 'foetus'.
Although it does not have a personal name it belongs to the
matrilineage of its previous human birth. Having changed in
this way the spirit child must make its way back to the
islands by drifting around in the sea; floating on driftwood,
leaves, dead seaweed and other light substances which litter
its surface. To ordinary people these spirits are invisible
although those able to go into a trance may see them and
fishermen may hear them calling 'wa wa wa' in the sighing
of the wind and the waves.

The spirit child is taken to the womb of a woman on the
islands by another spirit who is sometimes the ancestor of
the mother or father and about whom either of the parents
may dream. The ancestor spirit brings the spirit child to the
mother and puts it in her hair after which she may suffer
headache, sickness and a stomach ache. The blood from the

mother's body rushes up to the child and on the tide of this blood the child descends into the woman's womb. This blood then continues to nourish the baby which is why menstruation stops.

This explanation has aroused intense debate amongst anthropologists arguing whether or not the Trobriand Islanders were aware of the need for sexual intercourse before a baby could be conceived. At the time when these ideas were first collected, during the 1930s, the islanders had a somewhat hazy belief that sexual intercourse opened the way for a baby to be conceived although some believed that it was possible to become pregnant just by bathing in the sea where there was much seaweed and other debris on which the spirit babies might be floating. Like the Aborigines their explanation for the similarity between father and baby was explained by the father's close proximity to his wife during pregnancy and birth. Nowadays, the Trobriand Islanders are aware of the physical facts of conception and birth but this does not seem to have invalidated their spiritual beliefs about it.

Traditional explanations about how the baby develops encompass not only the visual physical changes, such as the cessation of menses and the growth of the baby, but also the baby's spiritual development. The Malay child is said to be formed first in the father's brain from where it travels to the father's eye and then to his chest. Here, within the dwelling place of the heart which is thought to be the microcosmic centre of the universe for each person, the baby experiences rationality and the father's emotions. From there the child descends to the father's penis and is thrust into the mother's womb. This is the baby's resting place where it grows and receives its mother's earth, air, fire and water until it is ready for birth. Until the fifth month the baby is thought to grow 'by the grace of God' and to share in its mother's soul so that if it is born before this time no Islamic burial is necessary as it is not an independent person.

On the island of Truk, in Micronesia, a baby is not considered fully human until after the mother's morning sickness has ended. If there is a miscarriage before that time then the baby was only a ghost, not a human being. In some places the period in which a baby is considered not completely human extends for a time after birth. On the island of Sulawesi in Indonesia, for example, Toraja babies who die before they have teeth are not given a normal burial but are put in the trunk of a special tree. God resides in the tree and because the babies are not yet fully human they can be given straight back to God without the need for a burial ceremony to smooth the path between earth and heaven.

The cessation of the menses is one of the first signs of pregnancy and in many places the blood which would have been the menstrual flow is thought to play an important part in the baby's development. Azande women in Africa say that during pregnancy a great amount of blood collects in the woman's body, within which is the tiny speck of the unborn child. As the child grows and changes into the form of a human being, the blood forms a net around it and comes out as the placenta after the baby is born. As the child grows it nibbles at the net with its lips and rubs it with its nose and it is these movements which the mother can feel and which make her groan if they are very fierce.

Amongst the Bavenda, another tribe in east Africa, the red elements of the child's body such as the blood and skin are thought to come from the mother, while the white elements such as the teeth and bone come from the semen of the father. Babies in Thailand are thought to start as hair but to be transformed into blood from which the baby's body is built. In the third month or so when the mother first feels the movements inside her, this is the *khwan* soul of the baby flitting in and out of the baby's heart.

In Sumatra, the Batek baby's *tondi* or soul substance originates while it is still inside the mother and its nature determines the future life of the person. The only way to improve one's lot in the world is to nourish and guard the *tondi* so that it does not leave. In many places the baby has more than one soul; for example, amongst the Karen a baby has thirty-three souls that dwell in various parts of the body. The six most important are in the eyes, nose, tongue and ears. Unlike many other places, however, these souls are not thought to come into the baby until the moment of birth and the evidence that they have attached themselves firmly within the baby is that the umbilical cord falls off without problem.

In Mexico the explanation of the baby's development also explains why a girl or boy is conceived. A male baby is formed from the nature essence of the mother and a female from the nature essence of the father. During sexual inter-course the mouth of the uterus opens and if pregnancy is to occur a drop of blood from either the father or mother falls and becomes the first substance of the embryo. If the first drop is from the father then the child will be a girl whereas if it is from the mother the child will be a boy. As the embryo grows it will migrate to its proper position within the womb – on the right for a boy or the left for a girl, with the placenta on the opposite side.

At first, when I heard such explanations I found it difficult to take them seriously and it was tempting to dismiss then as no more than primitive fairy stories. These explanations, however, have a far wider application than the narrowly physical focus of modern medical theories, encompassing as they do natural, social and spiritual forces.

For the modern doctor trained in western medical care, the process of conception, pregnancy and birth is perceived as primarily a physical one. This stems from the Cartesian idea of the distinction between the body and the mind/soul, that the body is separate from the mind and functions more or less independently of it. This medical approach, which is often called 'biomedicine' to distinguish its biological orien-tation, views the body as a biological machine, liable to malfunction from time to time either as a result of internal wear and tear or because of the invasion of external factors. 'Disease' has come to be seen as something which invades the ill person's body and which must be driven out before the sick person can be cured; as something separate which has to be got rid of rather than something which is part of the person as a whole.

Current knowledge of the body and its mechanisms is derived from systematic scientific study, much of which is undertaken in the laboratory. The efficacy of a particular treatment is similarly tested by using objective scientific techniques in clinical trials which remove the subjective bias of those providing the treatment. This type of medicine has, for some things, been successful beyond all expectations, especially in the treatment of infections and surgery, but much less so in the treatment of chronic conditions, particularly the scourges of modern civilization such as high blood pressure, heart disease and cancer.

This view of the nature of medicine, however, makes it harder to deal with the subjective feeling of illness and with psychosomatic diseases. A large proportion, variously put at between 50% and 70%, of all those who visit general practitioners go because they feel ill although no organic cause can be found for their illness. According to the biomedical view they are not 'properly' ill – however sick they may be feeling.

Health systems which are derived from more holistic concepts do not necessarily distinguish physical illness from other kinds of misfortune. Symptoms of any kind may be the result of physical, social, emotional or spiritual influences and will require different remedies to put them right. This might include herbal medicines, individual or social ceremonies or spiritual/magical rituals, although in most cases a combination of things will be specially tailored to suit individual needs.

Amongst people from traditional cultures, biomedical medicine is not necessarily considered superior to their own systems of medical care, sometimes much to the surprise and consternation of doctors attempting to introduce biomedical-type care in third world countries. I can remember a Karen man from northern Thailand telling me that the reason that western doctors had to use a lot of drugs was because they did not have access to magical and spiritual resources. Without these, the effectiveness of any treatment was limited to the properties of the ingredients used to bring about a cure, which in the case of biomedicine was mostly drugs. Traditional Karen medicine, in contrast, had in addition the strength of incantations used by traditional healers which had within them the power of every person who had learnt and used that incantation since its discovery centuries ago. Also, of course, in many third world countries biomedicine has the considerable disadvantage of being very expensive and centred in a few hospitals in urban areas. This makes it inaccessible for the poor and those in rural areas.

The biomedical approach has, however, provided us with more anatomical knowledge than ever before of how the unborn baby is conceived and grows physically within the womb. With the help of ultrasound and a range of sophisticated tests, the modern obstetrician can look at and monitor every stage of the unborn baby's growth and development. There is a wide range of techniques which can be used if things go wrong, from artificial conception and 'test tube babies' to the treatment of various conditions *in utero*, and surgical and other techniques when there are problems in giving birth. These represent considerable breakthroughs for the medical establishment and for the few women who have difficulty in having a baby. For the majority of women, however, as subsequent chapters will show, the physical focus of the biomedical care they receive has many negative effects.

Even in the most patriarchal societies, giving birth is the special concern of women; an area which is uniquely hers and in which she alone controls the decisions which have to be taken about it. In many cultures, pregnancy and birth are the primary arenas in which women have status and prestige which is denied to them in the society as a whole. Women of the Buu tribe in Africa, for instance, are entirely responsible for the birth process with women being solely accountable for the production of perfect children. Only women give birth and because it does not require a man's presence, men are forbidden both to see or discuss it.

If a woman has many unsuccessful pregnancies the women of the tribe will consult together to decide the reason for this. Perhaps it was the woman's fault because she was obstinate during delivery or committed adultery, or perhaps there was a man who in some magical or other way prevented the woman from successfully giving birth. Should a woman or

man by these kinds of actions 'kill a child' then the women
have the right to inflict various punishments on the offender.
Perhaps the most important (and painful) of these is 'pinch-
ing' when the woman or man will be pinched by all the
women of the tribe. Although a painful procedure, it also
has a therapeutic effect for any woman who has to undergo
it as she knows that afterwards she will be able to successfully
bear further children.

Giving birth, for the women of the African Benins, provides the opportunity to show endurance, stoicism and
impassivity in the face of pain and danger. Women who have
produced many children, especially sons, have considerable
respect and influence amongst the other women, for whom
they provide advice and help during pregnancy and birth.
Witchcraft is a possible source of misfortune and the detec-
tion of infants who may be witches requires vigilance.
Women therefore prefer to have a solitary delivery and will
only call for help perhaps to cut the umbilical cord and
deliver the placenta. This gives them the opportunity to diag-
nose possible signs of witchcraft in the baby and to take
appropriate action. What she decides to do with the baby is
a decision for the mother alone and no-one else, in particular
a man, is allowed to interfere.

In Guatemala, women are initiated into their roles through
their own experiences firstly of menstruation and then giving
birth. This is, however, not without its difficulties as there
are considerable barriers of ignorance and shame to be overcome and few women know or talk about these events prior
to experiencing them. A woman is usually unprepared for
her first menstruation, for her first experience of intercourse
and then the birth of her first child. She learns about each
mainly through her own body although she can seek the
help of other women, especially at birth when the midwife/
priestess will be called. Despite her ignorance and fear, each
experience admits her further into the female secrets shared
by other women of her group. Not only does she come to
understand her body, but also the cosmic forces which control life itself.

When talking to women from traditional societies, I was

always struck by how much giving birth was central to both their experience and identity as women. Deciding not to bear children was an unthinkable option as having a family was one of those things, like the sun and the rain, which was part of the natural order. This is not to say, however, that all traditional women feel that they have no choice in the number of children that they bear. I remember talking to a group of Orang Asli women, living in the jungles of Malaysia, whose attitudes towards contraception reminded me of my middle-class friends at home. They felt they could control their fertility with various herbal remedies from the jungle although none would have chosen to be childless. Pregnancy and giving birth were both central and normal parts of life and although the woman may have taken special care to protect herself and her unborn child, it was not a time of special risk. Things may go wrong, but most of the time they didn't, especially among groups which were well-fed and healthy. Birth was a family affair and took place within the family from whom the pregnant woman drew both her knowledge and her help for giving birth. All would participate in the birth process in different ways that reaffirmed for everyone whatever explanation they had about life on earth.

There could not be a starker contrast between this idea of the nature of the birth process and that which seems to be prevalent in the developed world. While for the mother in a traditional society giving birth is a part of normal life, in the west it is considered to be a medical problem fraught with danger and requiring the ministrations of professionally qualified medical personnel. Traditional women turn to their mothers and other female relatives for advice and help. In the west, the fast and ever-changing development of medical technology gives mothers very little to teach their daughters about birth. They must, as I did, turn to books and rely on the medical profession for information. Birth rarely takes place in the home, but in medical institutions where all the paraphernalia considered necessary to ensure a safe birth can be centralized.

The ideas of birth as both a physical process and a medical event which must be controlled and managed by

professionals (which have had such a profound effect on
obstetric practice in the west) are in the process of being
exported to third world countries. This, of course, is where
the holistic ideas about pregnancy and birth described in this
book have come from. When women with traditional medical ideas decide to have western-type obstetric care they must
cope with a new and different system of values. This has
been graphically described by Margaret Muecke[2] who compared the experience of traditional and modern hospital birth
amongst women in Chang Mai in northern Thailand. By
choosing to give birth in a modern hospital, women had to
accept the western medical definition of pregnancy as a medical problem to be controlled by more or less anonymous
specialists carrying out standardized techniques on those
parts of the woman's body which were relevant to the pregnancy. The woman had to present herself to medical specialists early in her pregnancy and to accept that it was an
individual problem for her that was separate from and did
not involve her family. The women in Chang Mai who had
a hospital birth were on the whole enthusiastic about it as
they thought it was safer to have a baby there, attributing
this to the doctor's esoteric knowledge, powerful medication
and equipment and the hospital emphasis upon cleanliness.
They sacrificed the close support of neighbours and family,
stuck out the loneliness of labour and birth in hospital and
what they perceived as the hospital staff's invasion of their
privacy to do what they thought was best for themselves and
their child.

In my experience I have found women from traditional
cultures much less enthusiastic about going to hospital to
give birth as often it is perceived as a place of loneliness and
invasive techniques such as induction and episiotomy. In
many places this type of care disrupts the strong cohesion of
women that grows from the shared experience of helping
with giving birth. Benin women in Africa who wanted to
give birth in hospital found that it diminished their responsibility and authority. They had to have their husband's per-
mission to go there and they lost their individual right and

ability to decide the fate of their child as well as the opportunity to gain prestige by a solo delivery.

Many would of course say that these are small things to lose for a safer delivery, but all too often there is only sufficient money to provide the minimum of physical care. Antenatal clinics are overcrowded and maybe only available in urban areas. The care for women giving birth is far more mechanistic than in the west as this is all that can be provided with the funds available. Traditional care and support systems are destroyed but only the worst of biomedical care is provided in its place. I think it is ironic that while in the west we are beginning to see the poverty of the totally physical approach to giving birth and to search for alternatives, in many third world countries their indigenous holistic ideas are being destroyed in favour of the biomedical approach.

Traditional explanations about where babies come from are often not anatomically correct but they place the events of birth in a much wider social and spiritual context than the narrow physical focus of the biomedical approach. They describe the reality of the intimate physical and spiritual relationship between the mother and her unborn child. This is a reality which is denied by the biomedical perception of the process, where birth is seen as no more than the physical extraction of a healthy baby and the mother no more than a vessel for the baby's development. This approach devalues and discounts the centrality of the mother's role in the birth process and the biomedical obstetric care that we provide for mothers is the poorer for it. In the west we are just beginning to understand how the physical process of birth is intimately dependent on psychological and environmental states. We are beginning to see how the process of giving birth can so easily be disrupted by the sorts of intervention favoured by a purely physical approach. More and more we are realizing that babies do not come from the body alone and that these traditional ideas, although we may not want to accept them in their entirety, have much to teach us in our search for a more holistic vision.

CHAPTER TWO

PREGNANCY

•

THE FIRST FEW MONTHS

Am I pregnant or not? A few women can answer this question with certainty right from the very beginning, but for most of us it is a matter of seeing the initial signs and seeking positive confirmation from some kind of pregnancy test. A few days after the cessation of menstruation (the first reliable sign of pregnancy), it is now possible to know definitely whether one is pregnant or not.

I never realized how much this changes the perception of becoming pregnant until I became pregnant for the third time while carrying out research in rural Indonesia. There were, of course, no pregnancy tests available so for the first few weeks and months all I had were the internal signs from my body. I was surprised how subtle these were and how my knowledge of being pregnant came very gradually, rather than all at once. As the signs multiplied, I felt my body changing and I became more certain. Like many of the women I was talking to, I went to a traditional Toraja midwife who massaged me and confirmed what had by then become obvious to me. I returned to 'civilization' before the pregnancy was apparent to everyone else and was amused to find that some friends doubted my certainty in the absence of a test. 'But how can you be absolutely sure?' one of them asked and it was then that I realized the extent to which we have come to rely on these external tests rather than our own internal knowledge.

I felt that the gradual awareness of my pregnancy was probably very similar to the way in which the initial stages of pregnancy are experienced by women in traditional societies. If they want further confirmation, however, there will often be some older experienced woman to whom to turn for help. Sometimes this woman may be known as the traditional midwife, implying either that she has some supernatural mandate for doing the work or that she has some special training acquired by working for many years with another experienced practitioner, usually her mother or other female relative. Traditional midwives live the same sort of life and do the same sort of work as the women they help. Unlike the modern midwife they see themselves only as a resource for women who need help, this being given according to the individual needs of their clients. They do not see themselves as a professional person who must carry out certain prescribed duties if they are to feel that they are doing their job properly. Women can turn to a traditional midwife for help at any time during pregnancy, labour and birth and the midwife will see it as her duty to respond. Often, however, women rely totally on the help of their female relatives and friends, only calling on the midwife if there are special problems or more expert assistance is required.

When I began talking to traditional midwives I was at first surprised at how little they were involved with women during pregnancy. Occasionally they would be asked to confirm a pregnancy and most of the women I spoke to were proud of their ability to do this during the early months, using massage in conjunction with other signs such as changes in the breasts and the feelings of the mother. Nearer to the birth, they might be asked to massage the mother and make sure that the baby was in the right position to be born. Apart from that they would only see women who felt they had problems; perhaps they were bleeding, were experiencing pain or had fallen down and were worried about the baby.

Although a pregnant woman might not consult anyone outside the family about the pregnancy, this did not mean, as it might in the west, that she was isolated without help and support. The woman within a traditional society has a close social network of relatives and friends and it is to these women that she turns for help when she becomes pregnant. In many cultures women, even when they become pregnant for the first time, will know a lot about giving birth from having watched other women do so and from having discussed it with their mothers. I remember talking to a Karen midwife who told me that of course every mother teaches her daughter about giving birth so that when the time comes she will know how to look after herself. Even in those places where a woman does not have this prior knowledge, becoming pregnant will signal her need for help from other women and thus she will gain access to the knowledge which women have to help them give birth successfully.

Pregnancy is normal but at the same time it is also a period of special vulnerability for both the mother and her unborn child. Pregnant women in traditional societies do not, on the whole, change their lives very much. Most of the mothers that I visited in south east Asia made few changes to their lifestyle and thought that if pregnant women carried on their normal work for as long as possible this was the best way of ensuring a trouble-free pregnancy and an easy labour and birth. In some cultures, however, pregnant women are thought to have special powers and are therefore restricted in some of their activities. Cherokee pregnant women, for example, are not allowed to cook for their families and in Guatemala the accumulation of blood in their bodies is thought to make them 'hot' and 'strong' and the intensity of their gaze enough to cause young babies, animals or plants to sicken and die.

Life may continue as normal but this does not mean that the pregnant woman does nothing to ensure that the pregnancy proceeds successfully to the birth of a healthy child. Not surprisingly, the measures undertaken vary considerably between different cultures although, as will become apparent, there are also a surprising number of similarities. Even within the same culture, however, there are often considerable differences between individual women who decide on different ways of looking after themselves. In many places there are special precautions that have to be taken with a first

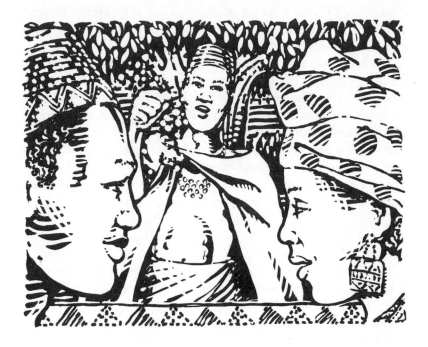

pregnancy which, if this is successful, will not be required for subsequent pregnancies. If a woman feels at special risk – perhaps she has had problems conceiving or trouble with previous pregnancies – she may feel that she needs to take more care and undertake special protective measures. She is concerned not just with the physical process but with how she can protect herself and her unborn child from harmful influences and how she can harness positive powers for her benefit. To look after herself successfully she needs to pay attention to emotional, social and spiritual as well as physical needs.

In many societies pregnant women are thought to be par-ticularly vulnerable to malevolent supernatural forces so when a woman becomes pregnant, various ceremonies are undertaken to ensure the safety of both herself and her unborn baby. In Africa, when a Ga woman becomes preg-nant her husband takes her at night to the tree of the family god. Here both are blessed and given holy water for washing and nyanya leaves to use as a sponge. These leaves are taken home, dried and kept until delivery. If the labour is long and/or difficult the leaves are soaked in water and the liquor given to the mother to drink.

Pregnant women are particularly susceptible to witchcraft so, with the help of other women, another ceremony might be undertaken to protect against this possibility. The pregnant woman has to wash herself in a bath containing a powerful herb and a large number of different sorts of food. The other women sit around suggesting various sorts of food which can be included and throwing small pieces of food into the bath. The idea is that however eccentric or catholic the witch may be in her tastes for things to eat she will find the food has been included in this concoction. The food in which the woman bathes protects her by saying to the witch, 'I am your own food; you cannot hurt me without hurting yourself'.

'Being taken to the water' is a ceremony that the Cherokee (native Americans) undertake on many occasions, the beginning of pregnancy being one of them. One aspect of this ceremony is the use of sympathetic magic in the bath which the woman takes before the ceremony begins. The way that such magic works is that items (which could be any animate or inanimate object) which have certain helpful characteristics are used magically so that the useful attributes are transferred from the item to the person. In this case the bath contains many herbs which include a mucilaginous bark from a tree to make her insides slippery so that the child will slip out easily, a herb to frighten the child and make him or her 'jump down (or be born) briskly' and two plants which are evergreen to impart longevity and health to the infant. She goes to the river, usually with her husband who acts as attendant for the priest, where she induces vomiting to cleanse all disease from her and the baby. She takes with her two white beads, symbolic of life, and two red beads, symbolic of success, and these will be put on the ground with a yard of white calico. The ceremony is undertaken by the priest to provide protection for mother and child as well as to divine the sex and health of the unborn baby. If negative influences are found further protective measures in the form of ceremonies and herbal medicine may have to be taken.

Harnessing the powers of important deities with prayers and offerings are in some places thought to be the best form of protection. When a Mayan woman in South America thinks she is pregnant she goes first to the midwife to confirm it. Once this has been done she goes to the church to light a candle and continues to do this on every following fifth day. Husband and wife should go together to do this on every twentieth day throughout the pregnancy. In Japan, once the pregnancy has been confirmed, the expectant father goes to the nearest shrine of Kuan Yin, the goddess of mercy, to pray for a safe birth and a healthy baby. This goddess is extremely popular amongst women in both Japan and China and is thought to help women with all problems to do with childbirth and children.

PROTECTING THE UNBORN CHILD

Mother and child are intimately connected; the unborn baby is completely dependent on the mother for its physical growth and, more importantly, for its physical and spiritual protection, while at the same time it is also growing into an independent person. Not surprisingly the mother, and to a lesser extent the father and other people in the pregnant woman's environment, is thought to have profound effects on her baby. These effects may be general in terms of qualities and characteristics which may be imparted to the baby, or they may be more specific in terms of particular things which the mother experiences or things which she does to produce a physical or other effect on her baby.

The general surroundings of the mother are thought by the Ga to have a considerable influence on the child. Women who live on high hills with a far-reaching view have tall robust children who don't feel the cold of the winds. Women who live on grassy plains (which in Africa are periodically burnt smooth and black) have smooth-skinned, very black children. Women living near the roar of surf and strong sea breezes have boisterous, loud-voiced children, and those who live near the sight of people battling with the waves of the sea, swimming, canoeing or wrestling in the water or on the beach have brave and vigorous children. People who live in the forest and are often startled by the echoes of chopping wood and trees falling down have timid, startled children. Like mothers in many cultures, Ga women believe that the talents and temperament of the child are affected by the ancestors, the linkage of grandparents, great-grandparents and so on that she can trace back to the origins of her particular tribe. The physical characteristics of the child, however, are affected by external influences on the pregnant mother. For this reason pregnant women should not look or play with an ugly animal like a monkey or pig as such hairy or woolly animals could make the baby look the same. If the pregnant woman wants to have a broad-faced son (which is considered very handsome) she should go and look at a broad-faced girl and embrace her frequently.

In Thailand it is thought that every sight, sound, touch taste or smell, every thought and action of the mother has some reaction on the child. She therefore takes every opportunity to associate herself with objects and people which have a positive effect upon the child and with words and actions which imply success giving birth. She does not, for instance, talk about or do anything which implies a blocking up, in case her body blocks up and the child cannot get out. She eats lotus buds which have been chanted over by a Buddhist monk so that her body will open up like a lotus flower and she will give birth easily. In Hawaii, whatever both parents do during the pregnancy is thought to affect the child. If they are busy and industrious in work then the baby will be the same and conversely if they are lazy and slothful.

Almost universally, pregnant women are encouraged to have as little as possible to do with illness, death and the dying. Pregnancy is, for the unborn child, a transitory state of vulnerability. Being not yet completely part of the living world the baby can suffer from the spiritual forces around those who are dying. In Ireland a pregnant woman should not enter a graveyard lest she turn her foot in a grave and cause her child to have a club foot. Palestinian pregnant women are told they should not walk in cemeteries and in Thailand pregnant women should not watch a cremation or visit people who are seriously ill. Amongst the Ozark people in the USA*, pregnant women should not look at a dead body as it could mark the child and might even, more seriously, cause a stillbirth. The Cherokee pregnant woman will not look at a corpse but if this cannot be avoided she must be the first to do so, otherwise she may have problems with giving birth. The Karen think that if a pregnant woman goes to a funeral the baby's soul, which has a very precarious hold on its body until some time after its birth, might be snatched by the departing soul and taken to the underworld.

The belief that lunar and solar eclipses can be very dangerous to unborn babies is found in many cultures in all parts of the world. It is perhaps hard to understand this when we know why they happen, but for people without this knowledge it must be a terrifying phenomena. It must look as if very powerful forces are at work with the possibility that the sun or moon, on which life depends, might disappear for ever. In the face of such powerful forces it is not surprising that those considered vulnerable, such as pregnant women, are thought to be particularly at risk of being affected. In Mexico, it is believed that a lunar eclipse might cause the baby to have an excess of parts such as extra fingers or toes. A solar eclipse might cause incomplete development such as a nose or ears incompletely formed because they have been 'eaten by the sun'. In Thailand, women used to believe that if they saw a solar eclipse the child might be born with a squint or to have a misshapen mouth resembling the eclipsed sun or moon. In these widely diverse places, however, the way to neutralize possible problems is the same: to wear metal, such as a safety pin, or to have a piece of metal under the bed.

* The Ozark people are descended from pioneers who came west from the southern Appalachians at the beginning of the nineteenth century and made little contact with the outer world for more than a hundred years. They come mostly from British stock and live in the Ozark country of Missouri and Arkansas and were described by Randolf in 1947 as 'deliberately unprogressive'.

There are many other physical phenomena pregnant women should avoid in case they leave a physical mark on the unborn child. In Ireland, for example, a pregnant woman tries to avoid meeting a hare to ensure that the child is not born with a hare lip. If she is unlucky enough to do so, however, she should tear the hem of her dress to transfer the blemish from her child. If she could catch the hare and tear its ear this would have a similar effect. In Thailand, mothers are very careful not to twist, cut or bang in nails as all of these might cause the babies to have deformities. If they chew betel leaf it is possible that the child may have an ear like a folded betel leaf. In Guatemala, some natural phenomena such as the sun or moon or thunderstorms may have an effect on the unborn child. Each of these natural forces is personified in a certain way and if the pregnant woman ventures out in the noonday sun, looks at the full moon or goes out in a thunderstorm there are certain physical effects, such as a club foot, which may result.

Unborn children are thought to be very sensitive both to their siblings and other unborn children. In Thailand, for instance, a pregnant woman should not watch another woman giving birth. The children in the wombs will be embarrassed by one another and refuse to be born easily. Amongst the Ga in Africa it is thought that the second child may talk to the first while he or she is still in the womb. If the elder child perceives that the coming child is of the same sex, it may become very jealous and this will be shown by it becoming greedy, bad-tempered, thin and ailing. A child displaying these symptoms is removed from the mother and sent to an aunt or grandmother.

I remember a Malay friend of mine telling me that when her third child was born the older sibling began to have very bad asthma. A *bomoh* (traditional doctor) was called and he diagnosed that the baby was jealous of the older child. He suggested that this was the cause of the asthma and that the baby should be sent away. My friend gave the baby to her sister to be brought up by her as one of her own children. From the time the baby left the house the older child's asthma disappeared and although she subsequently had more children, the older child never suffered from asthma again. In Mexico, if the child of a pregnant mother becomes ill and does not respond to normal treatment then it is thought that the jealousy of the unborn baby is the cause of the problem. Special ceremonies will be required to placate the unborn baby and persuade him or her to stop affecting the sibling in this way.

The effect of negative influences is increased if, as a result, the mother suffers from strong emotions such as fright or anger. Usually the effect is to mark the child physically or for the child to have some disability. An Ozark baby in the USA was born with a red mark on its cheek which was thought to derive from the experience his mother had of seeing a man shot while she was pregnant. As well as being very frightened, blood from the shot man had spattered on her face. This transferred itself to the baby who was born with a similar red mark.

In Europe, a baby's birthmark was thought to stem from the mother seeing something unpleasant or by being touched by some demon or evil spirit during her pregnancy. Often the birthmark would be in the shape of something that had frightened her, such as a dog or a gun. It was thought that the birthmark could be removed if the mother licked it. In Cambridge (England) a 76-year-old man once told a researcher of how his brother was born with deformed hands. His mother told him that when she was pregnant she had been alarmed by a dog which jumped up and put its paws on her stomach shortly before the boy was born. Because she was so frightened this experience imprinted itself on the baby in the form of the deformed hands which looked like dogs' paws.

This list of things which pregnant women should avoid might suggest that the pregnant mother in a traditional society goes around in a very fearful state, worried that her baby might be at risk from a wide range of negative influences. Carol Laderman,[1] who spent over a year in a traditional Malay village, found that this was not so. Although there are things that *may* attack the mother and unborn child and the mother needs to be aware of them, most of the time they do not and pregnant women can carry on their life as normal. Avoiding action, such as wearing a pin to negate the effects of an eclipse, can often be taken and even if not, women considered that they had a very good chance of remaining unscathed. Pregnancy and birth were normal events and although problems were possible, they usually proceeded without mishap.

Carol Laderman found that these explanations were used far more after giving birth as a retrospective explanation for any problems and for indications as to how they might be solved. One mother, for example, was troubled by her newborn's sickness until she remembered that towards the end of her pregnancy she saw a cat being sick. This provided her with both an explanation of her baby's sickness and an indication of what she needed to do to cure it. She took a little of the cat's fur, burnt it and fed the ashes to the baby who then recovered. In this village mothers were also well aware of the things that couldn't be controlled. A baby might be born dead or deformed and these kind of things were decided by Allah and had to be accepted as God's will. No-one was to blame and whatever a woman did while she was pregnant would have made no difference.

In the light of what we now know about how the unborn baby develops it is all too easy to describe such beliefs as no more than primitive superstitions. How can being frightened by a dog possibly lead to the unborn baby being physically damaged, especially when it happens late in pregnancy after the hands have been fully developed? How can the shape of a birthmark be caused by anything that frightened the mother? How can the mother looking at an eclipse have any effect on an unborn baby? Whatever their physiological inaccuracies, however, these explanations do affirm the intricate connections between mother and unborn baby which are true everywhere. Not surprisingly, most modern research has focused on the physical connections between them and although we are slowly unravelling how these come about, some aspects are as mysterious as ever. In many cases, the causes of physical abnormalities are unknown and when it comes to milder physical effects and less concrete factors, such as the baby's psychological development, our knowledge about this is very small indeed.

Physically the mother and unborn baby do not share a common brain, nervous or blood system. The main physical link between them is through substances in the blood which pass from the mother to the baby through the placenta. From the physical point of view the most important of these are the oxygen and food substances which nourish the baby and enable him to grow and develop. In addition, however, the baby also receives a large number of other blood substances, in particular the chemical messengers called hormones, the type and number of which are directly linked to the mother's emotional state.

Thoughts and emotions originate in the outer part of the brain called the cerebral cortex and derive from a mixture of internal thought processes and external situations and events. These are converted to physical sensations by the inner part of the brain called the hypothalamus which lies under the cerebral cortex. This part of the brain controls the endocrine system of hormones and the autonomic nervous system which controls bodily processes like breathing and digestion which take place without our having to think about them. Usually we are aware of the complex chain of events which follow from our desire to carry out some physical action, such as picking up a crying baby or speaking to a child, to actually doing it. We may, however, be more aware of our physical reactions to extremes of anger or fright; the racing of the heart, the feeling of heat and flushing of our skin and the change in our breathing. This so-called 'flight or fight' response is programmed into our bodies to provide us with extra energy and alertness should it be necessary to take immediate action to avoid danger.

Suppose, for instance, that a pregnant woman feels emotions such as anger or fright. This is registered in her cerebral cortex and relayed to the hypothalamus. Here these emotions are converted into physical sensations through both nervous activity in the autonomic nervous system and hormones which are discharged directly into the blood from various glands around the body. The heart beats faster, blood vessels and pupils of the eye dilate, breathing becomes faster and the whole body becomes excited, alert and ready for action should it be necessary. These physical reactions are a common response to all forms of stress although a woman is unlikely to be aware of them except in more extreme cases. This, of course, affects the unborn baby as the hormones which are produced during this process ultimately cross the placenta and enter the baby's bloodstream.

This suggests that if a pregnant mother suffers from a lot of stress and her blood is continually being flooded with these hormones then her unborn baby will also be affected in some way. It is, however, extremely difficult to demonstrate the nature of these connections satisfactorily; in particular to show precisely how different kinds and levels of stress can adversely affect the unborn baby. There are a very large number of variables which are very difficult to measure and determine their independent effects. What is stress for one person may not be stress for another or if it is, may not be felt so strongly, with consequent differences in the physical response between two people.

Determining the extent to which different levels of stress in the mother affect the baby is even more difficult. The baby may be more or less sensitive at different stages of development and there may or may not be crucial stages when the effect of the mother's stress is worse for the baby. The baby's own neurological make-up may vary, making him more or less generally sensitive to his mother's stress responses. Also, of course, many factors may interact because the stressed mother may not eat so well or feel that she must smoke or drink alcohol in order to cope. The effects of smoking and drinking on the unborn baby are well known but even here research has failed to show the independent effects of these factors.

Daphne and Charles Maurer[2] carried out a very careful analysis of a number of different research studies which aimed to show the effects on the baby when the mother drank alcohol while pregnant. They found that many studies had methodological flaws like failing to account for the mother's smoking or age, or questioning the mothers after birth about how much they had drunk months previously. They describe two studies which they consider to have best overcome these methodological difficulties but even here, the relationship between drinking alcohol while pregnant and giving birth to smaller babies was not clearcut. In one case the researcher had great difficulty in finding respondents who drank sufficient alcohol while pregnant, mainly because alcohol often makes pregnant women feel sick. This suggested that those who did drink were physiologically different from those who did not and it may have been this difference, rather than the alcohol *per se*, which produced smaller babies. In the second study where some of the mothers were very heavy drinkers, those who drank the most gave birth to very lightweight babies. Alcohol would seem to be the culprit except that it was unclear the extent to which the heavy drinkers were not taking care of themselves in other ways. The heavy-drinking mothers may have been less likely to follow dietary advice, have adequate sleep or exercise and it could have been these factors combined with the heavy drinking, not just the heavy drinking on its own, which gave rise to the low birthweight babies.

We cannot, on the other hand, conclude that drinking alcohol has no effect on the baby's development. It has been possible to show, for instance, that immediately after the mother has an alcoholic drink there are demonstrable effects on the unborn baby. Minutes after the mother takes a drink it enters her bloodstream and crosses the placenta to the baby. It depresses activity in her brain and spinal cord as well as slowing her reflexes and it seems there is a similar effect on the baby who also has slower reflexes until the effects of the alcohol wear off. The long-term effects, however, are very difficult to show and the authors conclude that there are similar problems with showing any links between other factors such as smoking and the baby's birthweight. So often such factors are connected with generally high levels of stress and with other influences like poverty, bad housing and malnutrition. To determine their independent and interactive effects on the unborn baby is very hard indeed.

If it is difficult to show the effects of these more measurable physical stresses on the unborn baby's development it is even more of a problem to show the effects of psychological stress and the ways this might affect the psychological development of the unborn child. Perhaps one of the strongest pieces of evidence we have that such stress might have an effect on the unborn baby is a Finnish study, carried out during World War Two. This showed that when the baby's father died before birth the child/adult was more likely to have later psychiatric problems. In some way the unborn baby must have been affected by the mother's stress but the exact way in which this happens has so far been very difficult to determine.

Often research of this nature assumes a simple causal relationship; the mother experiences stress of a certain quantity and type and this must therefore have a particular measurable effect on the baby. The unborn baby is, of course, totally dependent on his mother for his existence but he is at the same time also an independent being. Even inside the womb the unborn baby influences his own survival. His placenta produces many hormones which help to maintain the pregnancy and the processes of birth are started off by hormonal changes, some of which are instigated by him.

From early in the pregnancy, it seems, the unborn baby is an independent person who, whatever the arguments as to his spiritual nature, also produces these physical aspects of his own individuality. This implies that his experience of stress cannot necessarily be determined by his mother's experience. Most writers are quick to point out that some stress is undoubtedly good for the baby's development. Uncomfortable emotion forces him to focus attention on and become conscious of it and then try to do something about it, usually releasing his feelings by kicking or other movements. One theory puts forward the idea that the process of responding to stress is essential to the baby's psychological development. As the baby experiences different types of stress and responds to it this concentrates his attention. The subsequent memory trace produced in his brain, when it has been repeated several times, reaches a critical level and coalesces into the unborn baby's first simple concept of himself.

Once the baby is born the variety of stimulation that he receives makes it hard to isolate the effect of any one prenatal influence of this kind. The baby may be protected from stress by his immaturity as, although this means he will be easily hurt, it also means that he will be easily healed. The Maurers believe that because of his immature brain anything that happens in the womb will leave no more than a shallow impression on his mind and character. This, together with the stimulation that he receives after birth, means that the effects of prenatal influences are probably negligible, they conclude.

While I agree that it is very difficult, if not impossible, to separate and determine the influence of prenatal experiences it does not follow that they are insignificant. There is a question mark over whether the first memory traces are eradicated, as the Maurers seem to think, or whether they are the basis on which future character and personality are built. As a mother I find it difficult to believe that no trace of the experience is retained. Every mother can feel her baby reacting to external things like loud noises or music and to her internal states of anxiety, anger, happiness and joy. As mothers we know we are connected on many levels with our unborn child and perhaps women from traditional societies understand this better than modern researchers trying to demystify the connections in purely physical terms. It is a very mysterious interconnectedness which can perhaps only be described in its totality through poetry, music or art.

EATING FOR TWO

In a traditional society food is much more than just the physical nourishment expressed in terms of protein, fats and carbohydrates. Ideas about food inevitably include notions about which foods are the staple items in a diet and which should be eaten to maintain a healthy balance within the individual. Food is the basis of health, but when a person eats a certain type of food she takes in not only the physical nutrition but also less concrete characteristics from it as well.

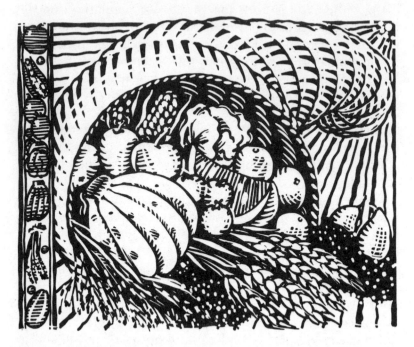

Thus, eating bananas provides carbohydrate and important minerals such as potassium; at the same time some cultures consider them cooling fruits which cool not just the body but one's anger and other 'hot' emotional states.

Not surprisingly, the food that a mother eats can have a variety of profound effects on her unborn baby. In Cambridge (England), for instance, a pregnant woman does not eat too many strawberries as this might cause the baby to have a strawberry birthmark. In Japan, pregnant women do not eat shrimps lest the baby be born with a crooked back similar to that of the shrimp. The Cherokee believe that eating ruffled grouse, raccoon or speckled trout will similarly mark the child and that no animals should be eaten that have been killed with bloodshed. The pregnant Thai woman avoids eating chillies in case they 'burn the baby's skin' whereas cooling bananas might be eaten to ensure that the baby has a cool temper.

It is also important for the pregnant woman to eat what she fancies otherwise this could be very bad for her unborn

baby. In Palestine, if a woman is deprived of food for which
she craves the child might have the characteristic of the food
on his or her body. A pregnant woman craved for a sheep's
head which she did not get and when her baby was born he
had hair like that of a sheep all over his cheeks.[3] A mother
might become swollen if she did not have the food she
desired; was this perhaps a sign of eclampsia, a condition
which may have some connection with an inadequate diet?
A similar belief amongst the Ozark stated that a child would
be marked with a birthmark or mole in the shape of the food
which her mother had wanted but had not been given.

The other possibility was that the child might become a
glutton for that sort of food. The Minangkabau from Sumatra say that a pregnant woman should be given what she
wants to eat otherwise the baby will be born with a lot of
saliva coming out of its mouth. The desires of a pregnant
woman for a certain food can overcome all other taboos
about how she should act and what she should eat. A Thai
pregnant woman craved a chicken which she killed herself.
This is normally considered a very dangerous thing for a
pregnant woman to do as killing a living animal could lead
to a stillbirth. In this case, however, it was felt that there
would be no negative consequences because she needed to
do it to nourish the child and this took precedence over
everything else.

In Hawaii, the food desires of a pregnant woman are
considered to be the wish of the child and to give some
indication of what the child will be like. If the pregnant
woman longs for *manini* fish this shows that the child will
be affectionate and as fond of its home as the fish, which is
very shy and timid and lives in sea pools. A longing for squid
means that the child will be clingy and will flee from anyone
that it doesn't like. A desire for *hila* fish means that the child
will be industrious and for tiger shark means that the child
will be a fearless fighter. If the mother vomits a lot during
pregnancy this shows that the child will be a good provider
– the mother can afford to get rid of food in this way as the
child will always provide more.

In the first few months of pregnancy many women suffer

from nausea and vomiting, although as one traditional midwife in Indonesia told me, this was to be welcomed as it
showed that the woman was really pregnant. Most women
agreed that this was something that just had to be accepted;
it would pass off eventually and there was no specific treatment. The juice of a young coconut was thought to be very
helpful and for those suffering badly this would be infused
with supernatural power from incantations and prayers said
by the midwife.

Certain sorts of food are eaten to ensure an easy delivery.
Minangkabau women, when they are pregnant, eat eel as
this is slippery and shiny and will help the baby to slip out
easily. Cherokee women do not eat squirrel in case the child
may lie in a humped position like a squirrel or 'go up' and
refuse to be born easily. Similarly, crawfish is not eaten as
this animal runs backwards and might encourage the child
to run backwards instead of forwards out of the womb at
the time for birth. The Yukaghir, a Siberian nomadic group,
believe that it is bad for pregnant women to eat the fat of
cow, reindeer or larch gum. They thicken or 'freeze' inside
and fasten the child to the inside of the womb. Butter from
the cow or horse's fat may be eaten as this melts in the
stomach and will help the child to slide out easily. In Hawaii,
in the months before the baby is born, the mother eats a
certain kind of blossom, the slippery juice of which is
believed to help as a lubricant for the birth.

These dietary restrictions have the social effect of setting
the woman apart from other non-pregnant women and
emphasizing her condition. As she is encouraged to ask for
what she wants, the pregnant woman has the opportunity to
get more of what she likes and wants than she probably does
normally. In many places women are the least well-nourished
members of the society; they are responsible for feeding
everyone else and must go short themselves if there is too
little food to go around. Often pregnancy is the only time
when a woman may have the chance to indulge herself and
whatever the other restrictions, pregnancy can be a time of
comfort and privilege with extra care and attention from
relatives as well as whatever extra food she feels she wants.

Traditional food restrictions during pregnancy and after are often condemned as being the cause of malnutrition amongst mothers and their newborn babies. Pregnant Yoruba women in Africa, for instance, are not encouraged to eat protein foods such as meat, fish or eggs which is the opposite of advice given to pregnant women in developed societies. In many places, such as Bangladesh, pregnant women are encouraged not to eat too much so that their baby will be small and more likely to be born without difficulties. It is easy to criticize these constraints, especially as they do not seem to conform to the idea of a healthy diet of sufficient protein, fats and carbohydrates that we have in the west. Often, however, critics fail to understand the underlying logic on which these strictures are based or to find out exactly what pregnant mothers do eat.

In too many places around the world, not having enough to eat is a fact of life either as a fairly permanent factor or as a possibility in certain years when the harvest is bad or fails completely. As previously mentioned, women are often the last to eat in a family and must go hungry when there is not enough food to go round. This malnutrition may have many effects on their bodies, in particular that their bones are ill-formed, with pelvic outlets, through which the baby must pass to be born, being very small or deformed. In this situation it is reasonable to try to have a small baby as the effects of having a large one, which can only be born with the help of surgery, would be devastating for mother and child in a situation where the necessary hospital facilities are not available.

Critics often have little idea about exactly what pregnant mothers do eat. The Yoruba woman may limit her intake of protein foods like meat, fish and eggs, but as every vegetarian knows, it is quite possible to be very healthy on a diet which excludes all these animal products. Unfortunately the research article I read on this subject,[4] while roundly criticizing these beliefs, did not examine in detail what pregnant Yoruba women did eat so it was impossible to say whether they were actually malnourished or not.

Carol Laderman carried out some very detailed research

on the diets of pregnant women in a Malay village. She found firstly that it was very important to look at their diets over a fairly long period. In the past researchers had often asked respondents what they ate either on the previous day or in the previous week. This was not necessarily a very good indication of the adequacy of their diet as a whole, which varied far more from day to day and season to season than most diets in the west. In this village there were pervasive and strongly held ideas about the sort of food that pregnant and newly delivered mothers should eat, but despite this there was considerable variation amongst individual women in the extent to which these guidelines were followed or not. Some followed them assiduously while others ignored them completely; they were, after all, only guidelines and women abided by them according to what they felt their individual needs to be. Carol Laderman found that the most important factor in whether a woman was well nourished or not was her economic position. Those who were poor were much less well nourished than those who were not, regardless of their indigenous beliefs and practices about food.

Every culture has staple foods such as rice, maize or beans which often have a religious significance because of their important food value and which are rarely excluded from a pregnant woman's diet. Humans manage to live healthy lives on very different sorts of diets and it is possible that we adapt to various sorts of food according to what is available. Pregnant women may therefore be healthy on diets which do not conform to what is considered a good diet in the west.

The whole question of food and how to ensure that every pregnant woman is well nourished is a large one which is outside the scope of this book to answer. As this short section shows, however, for women in traditional societies eating is far more than just taking in physical calories for physical nourishment. 'Eating for two' is eating in a way which provides mother and baby with good things relevant to spiritual and psychological as well as physical health. Eating properly helps with problems like morning sickness and ensures an easy delivery. Improving nutritional standards must be carried out in the context of these beliefs as well as taking account of economic and political factors relevant to how food is grown and distributed.

HARNESSING POSITIVE POWERS — CHARMS AND INCANTATIONS

In the name of God of triune nature, He is the Mighty Benefactor, Creator of all the powerful witches whom eye does not see and thought cannot conceive. Who knows what is before it is, before whom the angels tremble with awe, and whom the devils fear for His power. All things in Heaven and earth worship Him and He rules over all things.

Oh God, by Thy Mighty Name and Powerful Ann and the Beneficent Light of Thy Face, protect the bearer of this my charm — what is in her womb and who will drink from her milk — from the devilish, cursed karineh *[a sort of devil who might be born with the child and who inhabits the underworld] by the power of this magic square and what of Thy Mighty Name it contains.*

Pregnant women in traditional societies can do far more than just avoid negative and malevolent influences; they have various ways of harnessing positive powers which will keep away evil and ensure that the baby grows well and is delivered safely. The above charm is one that Palestinian women might have written out for them by a magician and wear throughout the pregnancy together with the following magic square:

Make it your charge, O Gabriel, make it your charge, O Mikhail, make it your charge, O Rufail, make it your charge, O Suriya, make it your charge, O Maniyal, by the power and might of the Mighty God, the Almighty and His blessed throne and His dazzling light to burn the cursed karineh *and cast her in the fire.*

Similar charms and amulets are found in many cultures, their

main objective being to defend against evil spirits and to
ensure a safe delivery. A similar type of amulet was found
in old Siam (now Thailand); this was a sheet of palm leaf
on which a magic formula was written. It was folded and
strung on cotton thread and put around the neck of a pregnant woman early in the pregnancy. As the pregnancy pro-
gressed it eventually turned black and after delivery it would
be taken off and kept in a jar with turmeric and other
delivery articles. These could be used magically if either the
mother or baby experienced problems in the time immediately after birth.

In Haiti, pregnant women can go to the priestess of the
vodun cult for a protective magic charm. She wears it around
her neck or around her waist to protect both herself and her
child against malevolent spirits or evil magic which might be
brought upon her by another person. She can also ask the
priest to divine which spirit will protect her unborn baby
and whether there is anything that her own protective deity/
spirit wants. If necessary, she will make offerings to this
spirit so that she and her child will be protected. Yoruba
charms are more prosaic and consist of symbolic weapons
such as a stone or penknife which are carried by a pregnant
woman whenever she goes out of the house, especially at
night when the spirits are more active.

Eagle stones were important amulets used by British
women during the seventeenth and eighteenth centuries.
These small actites (lapis acquilaris) are of a light brown
colour and were usually imported from the east. Being rare
and exotic and credited with magical powers, they were
greatly prized by those women lucky enough to own one.
Women wore them in little bags around their necks during
pregnancy to prevent miscarriage and then tied them around
their thighs during labour to ensure an easy delivery. Belief
in the magical power of the stones, as well as their name,
sprang from an ancient belief that they could only be found
in the nests of eagles. Despite the veneration and admiration
that these birds enjoy in many different cultures, being variously known as the king of heavens and bringer of storms
and thunderbolts, they were said to have great difficulty in

laying their eggs and were unable to do so without the help of this stone. As well as helping the eagle lay its eggs, the stone also had the power of preserving the nest from poison. Women in the UK also used a snakeskin as a pregnancy charm, this being thought to prevent miscarriages and make delivery easier.

There are some evil spirits who are particularly attracted to pregnant women and can attack them in their vulnerable state. Special ceremonies to placate or otherwise neutralize them may have to be undertaken. In Sri Lanka there is a spirit called the *kumara*; it pursues pregnant women, making them sick and causing a difficult delivery. The woman therefore prepares an offering consisting of a raw egg, a handful of unhusked rice, red flowers, powdered resin, betel leaf, a copper coin and sandalwood. This is put into a small unused pot, covered with an earthenware dish and suspended from a support made of coconut leaves in the room where the woman sleeps and will eventually give birth. Once the offering has been made a ceremony is undertaken at which an *edura* or exorcist points out the offering to the spirit. She then forms a solemn pact with the spirit with the purpose of gaining the spirit's favour so that she will not interfere and cause problems for the pregnant woman. If the birth is successful then a ritual will be performed at which further offerings will be made.

Gypsy women believe that excessive pain in childbirth is due to ill feeling on the part of demons, one of which was born as a crayfish. For this reason women do not consume crayfish while they are pregnant in case this angers the demon. They protect themselves, however, by wearing a sachet full of crayfish shells and stag beetles (who are kin of the same demon). This stops the crayfish attacking them as he will not attack his own kin.

Girdles are powerful amulets. In Japan, during the fifth month of pregnancy on the Day of the Dog or some other day chosen especially for its auspicious nature, a special sash or *obi* will be purchased. The pregnant woman takes this to the Shinto shrine to be blessed after which she wears it continuously under her outer garments for the rest of the pregnancy. It holds the baby firmly in place and stops it moving around too much in the womb. It also stops the baby from growing too big, thus ensuring an easy delivery. It also keeps the abdominal area warm and therefore, according to the tenets of Chinese/Japanese medicine, the mother free from illness. At the time when the girdle is purchased and put on for the first time, some families hold a small party for relatives and the midwife who will be in attendance at the birth. The sash is 8–10 ft long and made of red and white silk which are the congratulatory colours. When the child is born some families dye the white part of the girdle blue and make it into clothes for the child. It is also customary to borrow a girdle from someone who has had an easy delivery, the woman lending the girdle being known as the 'girdle mother'.

From the time of the Druids to the nineteenth century, girdles with supernatural powers were used by women in Britain. Often they remained in the same family for generations or they would be kept in a convent such as 'Our Lady's girdle of Bruton, which is red silk and a solemn relic sent to women travailing so that they will not miscarry in partu'.[5] Another girdle reputed to have belonged to Mary Magdalene was also kept in a convent and sent to women in pregnancy and childbirth as necessary.

THE ROLE OF THE FATHER

In traditional societies pregnancy is the time when a woman turns to her female relatives and friends; a time when bonds between women are reinforced and their unique part in the process of giving birth reaffirmed. It is often assumed that in traditional societies, because the activities of the women are paramount, the fathers play an insignificant part in the birth process. Male roles vary considerably but in no society is the man absolved completely from action which will help his wife give birth. In some societies he is present during delivery while in others he may be excluded from the birth but have to carry out important rituals afterwards, often connected with disposal of the placenta. In others he is totally excluded: after his wife has given birth he may not see her or the baby for a week or more.

During pregnancy fathers may, like their wives, have to keep away from all things to do with death and dying to make sure that the unborn baby is unharmed. The Cherokee father does not dig graves or help with a burial in case his child is stillborn. Thakur fathers in India must not become involved in anything to do with the dead such as offering grain to the dead or be one of those who carry a dead body to the crematorium. Like his wife, the expectant father must avoid things which could mark the child physically. The Cherokee father does not put dents in his hat in case the child is born with dents in his head and he should, like his wife, abstain from wearing a neck scarf and not linger around doorways to ensure that the birth canal is kept clear.

The Malay father's actions affect the baby more at the beginning of pregnancy than at the end when what the mother does is far more important. He should not kill wantonly and should be careful when chopping wood that he does not leave splinters which might mark the baby. From the seventh month onward, he should not cut his hair so that the placenta will not break up. In Sarawak, eastern Malaysia, fathers should not strike things, tie things tight or do any household work with a *parang* (large cutting knife). Since much of what the men do necessitates these actions he is excused, provided the work is absolutely necessary for life. Otherwise he may have to get someone with a non-pregnant wife to start the activity for him, as this negates possible harmful consequences. In Mexico, the father must not drink to excess otherwise the baby may be weak, deformed or stillborn.

If the Malay expectant father goes out at night he should return home by a devious route to trick spirits who might harm his wife and unborn baby. The Batak wife from Sumatra is likely to suffer from bad dreams which can indicate that she is being bothered by bad spirits and needs her husband's protection at night to ensure that the baby is not upset. He

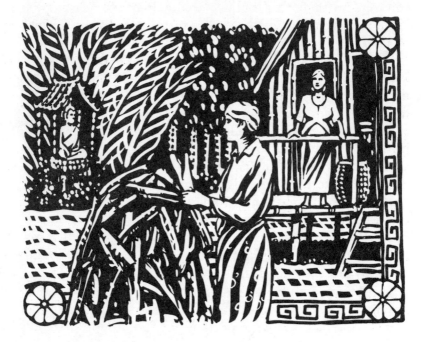

also goes out with his wife at night to protect both her and the unborn child from marauding night spirits.

In Thailand, the father shares responsibility with the mother for ensuring the safe pregnancy and birth of their child. It is his task to ensure that his wife is kept in a happy mood and to avoid quarrels so that they do not give birth to a quarrelsome child. During his wife's pregnancy he has to build a pile of firewood from *sahae* wood, a special kind of smokeless wood. A great deal of this is required and it must all be obtained from their land, although if this is not possible he may have to use other kinds of wood. The wood has to be piled in a certain way which is symbolic of the womb and must be covered with thorny branches to keep away the evil spirits so that they will not hurt the unborn baby. When labour starts he makes a hole in the pile, symbolically 'letting the baby out' and then pushes over the woodpile in the right direction (under the instructions of the midwife) so that his wife will give birth easily.

On the Pacific island of Truk, which is part of Micronesia,

the pregnant woman stays at home where relatives can care for her. The ideal husband tries to find any food for which she craves and is sexually true to her so that the pregnancy does not end in a miscarriage. This could happen if the wife even thinks that her husband is unfaithful so the good father will not do anything which might make her suspect his infidelity. In this culture, however, a husband is allowed to have sexual intercourse with certain other females during his wife's pregnancy although she must agree to this.

The couvade, in which the father suffers the symptoms of giving birth while his wife is doing so, has been discussed at length in the anthropological literature but in some cultures this starts long before birth. Ozark men joke about the way they often fall ill during their wife's pregnancy which, according to the wives, shows the depths of their husband's affection. 'My man allus does my pukin' for me', is how one Ozark woman described it. Ga women in Africa have a way of transferring any ill effects of their pregnancy to their husband. They step over his sleeping body during the night so that he can take on the discomforts of pregnancy. During their wives' pregnancies Ga men are often drowsy and lethargic while their women are full of energy.

The importance of sexual intercourse during pregnancy varies considerably. Amongst the Trobriands, for instance, the father's sexual intercourse is an important source of nourishment for the child. Similarly, the Ga consider that the baby is 'hatched' or grows with sexual intercourse; that it is good for the growth of the baby and helps the delivery. An Azande man, however, fears to have sexual intercourse late in pregnancy as he may spoil the child's mouth with his penis. In Truk, sexual intercourse, apart from possibly causing a miscarriage, may give the child a birthmark or a hare lip.

Many of these things, of course, ensure that the mother has, or can solicit, greater care and attention from her husband and emphasize the importance of her condition. At the same time, there may be social pressure on the expectant father to acknowledge her changed state and the effects this may be having on her and to do what he can to help protect

her and the unborn baby. Preparations that he has to undertake for the birth introduce him to his role as father as well
as establishing his new role with others, especially when it
is his first baby.

SEVEN MONTH CEREMONIES

Seven is a number with magical and spiritual significance;
by the seventh month of pregnancy it is usually well established and the mother is beginning to look forward to the
birth. In many places this is the time for a special ceremony.
Often this is carried out only during the first pregnancy so
that as well as protecting the couple and their unborn baby
and preparing them for birth, it also establishes the couple
socially in the status of potential family.

Sometimes these ceremonies can be quite elaborate affairs
as one was described in Java, the main island of Indonesia.
The ceremony is held at the home of the pregnant woman's
mother and includes much symbolic food. There is a dish of
rice for each guest which, being white on top and yellow
underneath, symbolizes purity and love. Rice mixed with
coconut and a whole stuffed chicken is given in honour
of the Prophet Mohammed. Seven small pyramids of rice
represent the seven months of pregnancy and eight or nine
round balls of rice symbolize the *walis* (Islamic saints) who
brought Islam to Indonesia. There will also be a large pyramid of a special kind of glutinous rice, thought to be very
sustaining; the pyramid made of it will be very 'strong' and
make the child strong also. Food from above and below the
ground symbolizes the earth and sky, and three kinds of rice,
coloured white, red and a combination of both symbolize
the mother's water (white), the father's water (red) and the
mixture of the two which has resulted in the child. There
will also be a very spicy food called *rujak legi* which the
mother will eat to determine whether she is carrying a boy
or a girl. If it tastes hot and spicy then she will have a girl
whereas if it tastes flat she will have a boy.

The midwife who has been asked to attend the delivery

takes an important part in the ceremony. The woman ties a
string loosely around her middle or holds a leaf in her hand.
The midwife has to cut off the string or cut the leaf in half
while chanting:

> *In the name of God, the Merciful, the Compassionate*
> *My intention is to cut open a young unopened leaf (or*
> *the string)*
> *But I am not cutting open a leaf*
> *I am cutting the way open for a baby to emerge*
> *I limit you (the baby) to nine months of meditation in*
> *your mother's womb*
> *Come out easy, go out easy*
> *Easy, easy, by the will of Allah*

Two green coconuts are then placed in front of the husband
and he slashes at these with his knife. If both split then it
will be an easy birth and if one splits then it is possible to
tell the sex of the child. If neither splits then the birth will
be difficult. Dropping an egg down the woman's sarong to
make it break and breaking a water jug by throwing it
outside are added ways of symbolizing the opening of the
mother's body and therefore bringing about an easy birth.

I came across a similar but less elaborate ceremony
amongst the Bataks of Sumatra. Here, during the seventh
month (and occasionally later) of the first pregnancy the
couple invite close relatives to a party. The couple sit together
and fish is brought to them as a present and nowadays often
money as well. Someone, usually one of the parents, takes a
Batak scarf and puts it around both of their necks and wishes
them a safe and easy delivery of the child.

The Pandits of India have a special ceremony during the
seventh month of pregnancy which is called the 'giving of
the milk'. At this time the pregnant woman goes back to her
parents' home for a few weeks. She comes back with gifts,
especially yogurt, which is distributed by her mother-in-law
to various members of her husband's family. Of particular
importance is the distribution of the yogurt as this ensures
the flow of the mother's milk to the child after birth. As well
as the symbolic meaning of this ceremony, which is to ensure

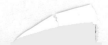

a safe birth, it also gives the pregnant woman a physical and psychological rest with her own family – very important when this is maybe the first time she has seen them since her marriage. It also provides a public announcement of her first pregnancy.

The Ga father of rank has an elaborate ceremony which involves both the priests and all the other (usually upper class) men of the town who have undergone a similar ceremony in their youth. To begin with, the man goes to the house of Na Yo, the goddess of birth, where he will be given a sacred hat decorated with gold which has been prepared by the priest. He puts it on and goes about the town visiting all the other men who have undergone the ceremony in the past, to give them money. For the next three days he stays with his wife but continues to wear the hat at all times. After this period of seclusion there are various ceremonies which include rubbing his body all over with a soft white stone to take away evil and shaving his head except for a tuft on top to which a gold coin is fastened.

Three days after these ceremonies the man puts on new clothes and revisits all the families to whom he originally gave money and receives double the money in return. Three days later he puts on his sacred hat and goes to the tree where sacred dances are held. Here the elder women of the town bring him various presents and his friends 'treat him as a chief'. They do this by raising him three times towards the sky and he is then taken to all the houses of the gods in the town. From then until his wife delivers he wears only white calico.

Once the child is born the last part of the ceremony is enacted. The man goes back to the priest of Na Yo who blindfolds him and shaves his head. He must not see the shorn hair which is stuffed into his hat and which he will not see again until he is dying when it will be put on his naval and buried with him. After the shaving he goes to thank his wife for the child and gives the child a present of money and white calico. This is used for the baby's pillow and a piece is always kept carefully. If the child later seems to be growing up to be disreputable, he will be shown this piece of white cloth to remind him that he was 'born in purity' and must not therefore carry out actions which disgrace his honourable birth.

ANTENATAL CARE

All this seems a very long way indeed from the experiences of pregnant women in the west. The majority of such women receive antenatal care from hospital clinics although it must be remembered that, worldwide, only a third of women giving birth have this type of care that we now consider as normal. Such care is, however, a very recent innovation. Only 200 years ago in Great Britain, women looked after themselves during pregnancy much as women in traditional societies do today. Until the eighteenth century, pregnancy was hardly thought of as a subject worthy of medical interest. Most women looked after themselves and gave birth with the help of other female relatives or midwives. Only the very rich could afford a doctor whose ministrations were usually confined to advice on lifestyle, abdominal palpitations and bloodletting which was the only treatment available to deal with and avoid complications. The conscription of men into the army for the Boer War in the late nineteenth century showed how large a proportion of the population was unhealthy and focused political attention on ways to better the health of the nation. It was then that the idea of antenatal care was conceived.

At different times, antenatal care has consisted of many different types of screening procedures and treatments. At first this was provided in the community by general practitioners and local authority clinics although in the last twenty years it has been centralized in hospitals where most births now take place. Women are encouraged to attend the antenatal clinic as early as possible in the pregnancy and to have a series of standardized tests of blood, urine, blood pressure, ultrasound, and in some cases amniocentesis, which will determine whether there are any genetic problems (in particular Downs syndrome) in the developing baby.

Advocates of antenatal care say that only by coming to the clinics early in pregnancy and submitting to these tests on a regular basis will problems be identified and dealt with early so that the mother will remain healthy and have a healthy baby.

Anyone who has spent hours sitting on the uncomfortable chairs of a hospital antenatal clinic, eventually seeing a rushed and harassed doctor for a very few minutes, cannot help but wonder whether this is really true. Research shows that many women are dissatisfied with the care that they receive and complain that it is too impersonal and mechanical as well as being highly inconvenient. Mothers must often travel long distances to centralized hospitals which have few facilities for younger children while they wait long hours to be seen by a doctor. Such complaints tend to be dismissed as doctors argue that any inconvenience is worthwhile if it results in healthier mothers and babies.

But does antenatal care as it is presently organized achieve this goal? If one looks at the history of such care one of the most disturbing things is the extent to which various procedures and tests have been introduced without adequate clinical evaluation and which have subsequently been found to be useless or dangerous. X-rays used to be used widely, drugs like thalidomide and DES were given to pregnant women, and despite the almost universal use of ultrasound, its long-term effects have never been properly evaluated. There has never been a randomized controlled trial of antenatal care; its advocates have always assumed that it is a good thing without any real experimental evidence for their views. Some evaluation has been carried out, however, although this suggests that the antenatal care which most women receive may not be quite as good as experts would have us believe.

Three of the most common problems of pregnancy are intra-uterine growth retardation (when the baby does not grow properly in the womb), pre-eclampsia (when the mother suffers from high blood pressure, protein in the urine and swelling in the tissues and which can lead to eclamptic fits with possible death of mother and child) and foetal malpresentation (when the baby is in a position which could make birth difficult). One important aim of antenatal care is to identify women with these common problems and give them prompt and effective treatment. Research in Aberdeen,[6] however, suggests that antenatal clinics may not be particularly good at doing this.

The researchers looked at the records of 1907 women who had delivered babies in 1975 and for whom complete records were available. They found firstly that risk prediction is very difficult as half the women whose babies died at or soon after birth had no risk factors at all. Only 44 per cent of cases of retarded intra-uterine growth were correctly identified before delivery and there was a very high false positive rate – 2.5 cases of incorrect diagnosis for every correct one. Only 1 per cent of pre-eclampsia was diagnosed before 34 weeks of pregnancy and 30 per cent of cases did not occur until the woman was in labour or post-natally. The number of women correctly diagnosed with pre-eclampsia antenatally was about the same as those wrongly diagnosed – 50 per cent of those diagnosed as having this problem were later found to have a temporarily raised high blood pressure which subsequently returned to normal. The identification of breech presentation was much better as 88 per cent of such babies were correctly diagnosed prior to delivery.

Obviously the productivity of antenatal care, in terms of identifying and treating common problems, is much lower than many doctors would like to admit. Despite this, however, advocates of antenatal care say that the cost is worth it if at least some problems are identified and successfully treated, however few these might be.

Aside from the economic cost there is, to me, the much more important but less quantifiable social cost of submitting large numbers of basically healthy women to medical screening. Firstly, the more screening tests that one uses the more likely one is to find abnormalities, even in apparently normal and healthy women. Often doctors may not be able to determine the significance and effects of so-called abnormal results and may end up provoking anxiety without being able to provide reassurance. The widespread use of amniocentesis, for example, has led to ambiguous diagnoses where the results are not obviously abnormal but are not completely normal either, and where the implications for the unborn baby are impossible to predict. The research in Aberdeen showed that for some conditions there were a very large number of 'false positives' which again must have provoked a considerable amount of anxiety for the women involved who may have suffered, as it turns out, for no reason at all.

Obviously doctors are not infallible, but the Aberdeen research did seem to show a very large number of incorrect diagnoses on women who were not sick but pregnant. Doctors may dismiss such anxiety as being irrelevant but it seems ridiculous that a so-called system of care provokes such a lot of this uncomfortable emotion so unnecessarily. The results of such anxiety have not been evaluated but at a time of such vulnerability and change, it can only make things more difficult.

Secondly, doctors tend to look for and emphasize the abnormal side of pregnancy and to expect problems rather than support women in having a normal birth. As any woman knows, being labelled 'high risk' according to factors such as age, about which one can do nothing, does not boost confidence and can turn into a self-fulfilling prophecy. Too often a visit to an antenatal clinic, rather than being a reassurance, is a threat to self-confidence, especially as doctors like to give the impression that pregnancy and birth are not safe without their ministrations. During my last pregnancy I always came away from the hospital antenatal clinic feeling diminished and depersonalized and I know that my experience was not unusual. I could not help comparing it with my feelings when I left the traditional midwife when I felt empowered and positive.

Antenatal care does identify and successfully treat some problems, but in doing so it often destroys the confidence that women have in themselves to give birth successfully. The pregnant woman in a traditional society takes total responsibility for the health of herself and her unborn baby. She is not alone, however, and asks for and receives care as and when she needs it from women relatives and friends.

They provide her with a variety of physical, emotional and spiritual support tailored to her individual needs that boosts her confidence in her ability to protect her unborn child and eventually give birth.

In contrast, women in the west are encouraged to rely on medically qualified doctors for their antenatal care which is usually provided in the relatively impersonal environment of the hospital clinic. Women are expected to attend the clinic on a regular basis whether they feel that they need to or not. The pregnant woman is encouraged to rely on the doctor's assessment of the baby's growth and development which is determined by various tests, especially ultrasound. It is the doctor's responsibility to find and treat any problems and the pregnant woman is expected to defer to his (and it usually is 'his') knowledge and expertise. Doctors tend to focus on the problems of pregnancy and are inclined to treat the normal processes of birth as a medical emergency which can only be solved with medical intervention. For a woman who expects to have a problem-free pregnancy this type of care can come as a rude shock, making her feel sick and powerless instead of healthy and empowered as she might have done at the beginning.

Modern antenatal care may identify and treat the problems of the few, but in doing so it often destroys the confidence of the many who have no problems and do not need any medical care. As we will see later, this has very significant implications for the way in which we now give birth in developed societies.

CHAPTER THREE

GIVING BIRTH

•

TRADITIONAL ANTICIPATIONS AND MODERN BIRTH PREPARATIONS

When I talked to pregnant women from traditional societies, their happy vagueness about when the birth was likely to take place always amused me. After my own experiences with modern doctors who provided a specific 'B-day' and started to worry once the baby hadn't arrived by that date, the relaxed attitude of these women was a tonic. They usually knew within a month or so as to when the baby might arrive and trusted to their own internal knowledge and experience of the pregnancy as to when birth would take place. In their own minds they made no distinction between the means they used to ensure a successful pregnancy and those they took to ensure an easy birth, although inevitably some of the things they did focused more on birth than on pregnancy.

To give birth, a woman must allow her body to open and to release the child. In the west, preparations for this usually include various physical exercises whereas in traditional societies women prepare more by symbolically clearing the way, a process which is often described as sympathetic magic. They avoid all thoughts and actions which have anything to do with becoming stuck or closing up in case this is transferred to their body and the child becomes stuck or their body refuses to open easily to give birth.

A very common action of this type, which I came across again and again in my travels throughout south east Asia, was the behaviour of pregnant women in connection with entrances and exits to houses. Malay, Minangkabau and Batak pregnant women avoid sitting in the doorway of their house or on the steps leading up to it in case this should cause a blockage and the child finds it difficult to be born. Thai women are very careful not to stop when ascending or descending stairs for the same reasons. Malay pregnant women are also careful to go out of a house by the same door that they came in, as 'there is only one entrance to the body' by which the child must come out. The Minangkabau pregnant mother, once she has started out towards the river to bathe, will not retrace her steps for any reason as this might cause her baby to turn back causing difficulties at birth. This is also found in other parts of the world; the Cherokee never loiter near doorways but pass through them briskly so that the child also will 'jump down quickly'.

To enable her body to open easily the pregnant woman should not do anything or place herself in a situation which implies a closing up or the making of an obstruction. In Thailand, for example, pregnant women do not sew up the ends of mattresses or pillows as this might cause an accidental closing up of her body. If a pregnant woman from the Karen tribe is out walking and someone fells a tree or accidentally puts something in her path, this could cause her body to become blocked up. To ensure that there are no harmful consequences, the offending person must give the woman a chicken in recompense. A pregnant Yukaghir woman in Siberia makes sure that no one crosses her path when out walking. She also raises her feet high and kicks away any lumps or stones in her way, symbolizing the removal of obstructions at childbirth. Like the Minangkabau, when she sets out for a place she does not turn back so that her birth will not be checked in the middle. Towards the end of her pregnancy her husband and relatives also perform these actions to ensure an easy delivery for her.

In many places the wearing of belts and neckerchiefs is discouraged, to prevent knots and kinks in the umbilical cord, or the cord getting wrapped around the baby's neck during birth. Cherokee women do not wear a neckerchief or belt of cloth during pregnancy and neither do they tie aprons around their waist in case the umbilical cord twists around the baby's neck. In Hawaii, women do not stitch together the materials used for roof and housebuilding or work with cords in case the kinks are transferred to the baby's umbilical cord. In Sarawak, pregnant women avoid tying things together with rattan although this is a job that often has to be done. If a job of this nature is absolutely essential, they find some non-pregnant person to start the job which they then finish, so that possible negative consequences are neutralized.

In traditional societies, it is generally believed that women who work hard are more likely to have an easy delivery; this is not only because it keeps them physically active but because it keeps them, and therefore the baby, 'loose' so that it will be born more easily. In Guatemala, a woman who fails to clean her grinding stone or tie her loom promptly will have a lazy child who, when birth is imminent, will be too slothful to be born easily. In Thailand women believe that hard work keeps the womb loose and thus prevents the child from becoming too big and fat and causing a difficult delivery. In Hawaii, every time a woman bathes she should move her abdomen to and fro so that the baby doesn't 'stick' and have a difficult birth.

Walking under the belly of a camel is, throughout the Arab world, believed to help a woman have an easy delivery. In Thailand a woman should walk under the belly of an elephant, especially if it has a kindly disposition. This is considered a generally lucky thing to do and now that few elephants are used in logging many of their owners bring their animals into the cities so that people can do this. Passing through a tunnel formed by shrubs and trees or going through the iron hoop used on barrels is how Swedish women ensured an easy delivery.

Birth preparation in the west is much more physically based, with various breathing and other exercises forming a large part of what is taught in antenatal classes. The roots of modern birth preparation stem from the work and writings of Grantley Dick Read whose first book on the subject

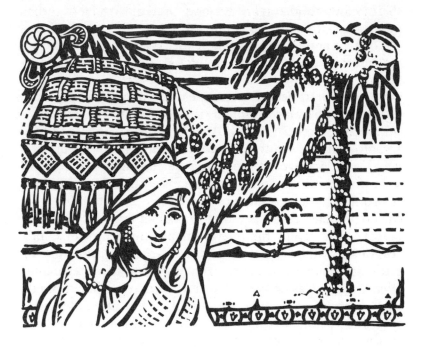

was published in 1944. He felt that labour pain arose from
socially induced expectations about pain but that it was not
necessarily an inherently painful process. He thought that
fear of childbirth led to it being very painful, the pain producing tension which affected the circular muscle fibres at the
bottom of the uterus, making it more difficult and painful
for the uterus to open. Such pain could therefore be elimi-
nated by firstly providing information about labour and birth
and correcting these misapprehensions. At the same time,
a series of breathing and other exercises provided muscle
relaxation which would lead to an easy and pain-free birth.

Another pioneer of modern childbirth preparation,
Lamaze, used the work of Russian researchers who claimed
to be able to block the pain perceptions of women in labour.
Performance of certain acts, mainly deep breathing, stroking
sections of the abdomen and stimulating the small of the
back, would create what was called a zone of 'negative induction' in the brain which blocked the incoming pain perceptions. Women were taught to stimulate their bodies and thus

their brains in the same way so that during labour their perception of pain was diminished.

Looking at the history of these ideas and how they became incorporated into modern antenatal classes, it is perhaps surprising to learn of the considerable controversy they provoked amongst medical personnel. Grantley Dick Read was charged with unprofessional conduct and was refused a permit to practise in South Africa, while in America obstetricians were for many years contemptuous of what the process could achieve. Perhaps not surprisingly, women and later their menfolk took to the process with great enthusiasm. It promised not only the possibility of a pain-free birth but that a woman could actually do something for herself to achieve this rather than rely completely on medical professionals. One doctor[1] wrote with great surprise that his patients seemed to want to carry on using these techniques even when it was obvious that they were not eliminating the pain. 'I have to persuade them to take medication', he writes in wonder, not realizing that some women prefer the pain to the effects of such medication in terms of the feelings of loss of control and responsibility.

Initially at least, antenatal classes provided mothers with a system of breathing, thinking and relaxing which was characteristic of a pain-free state. During classes women were taught how to enter this state at will so that during labour they could block off painful sensations. This skill was equated with other physical skills such as swimming, writing or even reading; something that one could control with the conscious mind. As one doctor[2] wrote: 'It is our impression that conditioning a woman for childbirth does very much for her what military training does for a young soldier who must face the rigors of battle. . . . with military training he becomes so conditioned that he is able to face death and pain with fortitude and to come through the experience with a sense of having proved his manhood.' Warming to this theme he then goes on to say how in the process of giving birth women can prove their womanhood: '. . . . what might we not achieve if we could persuade women to prepare for pregnancy and labour with the care that we train our young men for war or even with the care that a prize fighter gives to preparing for a fight.' The emphasis was on preparing women to control their responses and thus control their bodies. Those unable to do so were often described in pejorative terms as having insufficient self-control, being insufficiently trained or as not having the necessary will or backbone to carry out the exercises properly.

Initially, in France at least, the teaching was conducted by a specially trained woman called a *monitrice* who not only carried out the training but accompanied each of her pupils into the hospital and stayed with her until birth had taken place. One writer felt that such women 'were the key factor in the success of this form of labour management.' I think he was probably right although this may have been because of the individual support and attention that she gave rather than the training *per se*.

As antenatal classes became more widespread, both in hospitals and (in the UK) through voluntary associations like the National Childbirth Trust, this function began to be taken over by the father. He was increasingly allowed to be with his wife in hospital during the actual birth and, as it was usually impossible to provide a specially trained person to accompany every woman wanting to use this method, her husband took over this role. In much of the literature he is called the 'labour coach', his role being to keep his wife focused on her breathing and other exercises and acting as a mediator between her and the hospital staff. Again, however, there is the assumption of deliberate control, that the husband is helping his wife control the process of labour. The extent to which he, in this position of 'coach', is also controlling his wife in the vulnerable state of labour is rarely questioned or discussed. Usually on the basis of little or no evidence, it is assumed that this situation provides a more satisfying experience of birth for both of them.

How successful is this sort of preparation for giving birth? This is actually very difficult to show and in fact antenatal classes seem to be yet another of those things which have been brought in as being a 'good thing' without any proper evaluation. There is a difference here, however, in that the impetus for this sort of preparation has come from women themselves, often in the face of hostility from the medical profession.

Part of the difficulty in carrying out any sort of evaluation exercise is that the women who were the greatest enthusiasts for this process were not typical of the population as a whole, being mainly middle class and well educated. With their commitment to this process of birth preparation, it would have been difficult to assign them randomly to different groups and compare outcomes, which is the only way of scientifically validating the procedure. This, to my knowledge, has never been done in the pregnancy context although more general research on pain perception has been carried out which shows that the breathing and focusing techniques do have some effect on reducing perception of experimentally induced pain.

A recent research project,[3] however, which looked at the extent to which sixty labouring women found the process useful in coping with actual labour, was not very positive. All the mothers had attended hospital antenatal classes and had been taught a variety of breathing and postural techniques but by the beginning of the second stage less than a third of mothers were using them. A substantial number of the remaining two-thirds had epidural analgesia and few continued using these exercises once this had been administered. Over half of those not having this analgesia, however, carried on throughout the rest of their labour without using the techniques as they had been taught. Unfortunately this research was not detailed enough to understand why this should be so, although given the very large number of possible variables, the answer is unlikely to be simple. Was it the quality of the antenatal classes or was it something to do with the environment of labour, or did some mothers perhaps have more pain for which the coping skills were ineffective?

Modern antenatal classes and those who promote and provide them are perceived as firstly providing accurate information about birth and what is likely to happen in labour, as well as training in relaxation and breathing techniques. Here, the knowledge that in traditional societies is held by all women is removed from the female community and packaged as 'expert advice' which must be provided by professionals. All too often, however, and especially when they are based at a hospital, antenatal classes are no more than a forum in which women can be told about the advantages of technology and how it will be used, and getting them to accept the technological approach. I remember my own experience of these classes which, although providing exercises and discussion, also included a tour of the hospital equipment and long descriptions of when and how it would be used.

The exercises are often seen as providing women with more autonomy, usually meaning more chance of controlling her own labour with less likelihood of medical intervention, but often there is an assumption, sometimes unspoken but maybe explicit, that they are only of use if 'everything is normal'. Whether this is the case or not is determined by the doctor who may have an idea of an 'ideal type' labour, often expressed in terms of how long each stage should last. When labour does not proceed according to this prescribed timetable, the woman is expected to defer to the doctor and accept whatever intervention he deems necessary. For many women the knowledge that their labour must go according to a prescribed plan otherwise intervention will be used must inhibit their confidence and ability to give birth successfully. There is also often a very strong message that a woman must 'do what the doctor says' and in the beginning obstetricians would only support antenatal classes if this was accepted and made plain to the participants.

Or Michel Odent[4] thinks that this whole approach is the wrong one to prepare women for birth. Stemming as it does from the biomedical view of the body as a machine, it encourages the woman to think she can control the process in the same way that she controls her body in other physical activities like swimming. Giving birth, however, is under the control of the hypothalamus, the much more primitive part of the brain which controls our unconscious processes. Odent thinks that, to give birth successfully, a woman needs to yield to these primitive instincts deep inside her and let them dictate her physiological responses. This, he says, is the only way to attain the deep relaxation that enables a woman to give birth with the normal efficiency of other animals.

Thus, the way to prepare for birth is not to focus on physical means of control but to get in touch with and learn to trust our primitive and intuitive instincts. Research has shown that this primitive part of our brain can be accessed with the use of images and that images are potent ways of influencing it and the bodily processes that it controls. When the woman from a traditional society uses images to symbolically clear the way for her baby to emerge, she may well be acting on her hypothalamus and ultimately the process of birth itself. This may, in the end, turn out to be a much more potent preparation for birth than the exercises and breathing which are presently being taught in antenatal classes and which, by all accounts, are not as successful as their advocates would like to think.

THE MANY FACETS OF LABOUR

When I first began talking to traditional midwives about how they helped women in labour, it soon became very clear that what I meant by labour and what they meant by labour were rather different. I thought of labour as being in three stages: the first stage when the cervix opens, the second stage when the baby is born, and the third stage when the placenta is delivered. Thus, my idea of labour was just that, an idea of a physical process to which individual labouring women more or less conformed.

My respondents took a much more concrete view; women experienced labour in as many different ways as there were individuals to experience it. They found it very difficult to talk in generalities, preferring instead to talk about individual cases and concrete situations. There were general principles, of course, but the most important thing for these practitioners was to respond to the needs of the labouring woman, which at times could mean that they didn't follow their own general principles as they had explained them to me. When talking about labour they tended to focus spontaneously on what we call the second stage, when the baby is actually born. The rest of labour merged imperceptibly with ordinary life and was far more idiosyncratic, particularly in terms of the extent to which individual women needed and asked for help at this time.

I feel that any attempt of mine to write about labour in this context as a process which happens in different stages, or to try and separate different aspects of it, is to impose an order on it which in the minds of these women does not exist. Labour and birth is a time of maximum vulnerability; the help a woman needs at this time depends not only on what is happening in her body, but how she is experiencing it and the supernatural forces that may be helping or hindering the process. Every woman is different and the expertise of these traditional midwives lay in their ability to muster all their expertise at all levels in response to the woman's individual needs.

In many places there are special ceremonies which are undertaken either very close to the birth or when labour starts which will help to facilitate delivery. In Tikopia in the Solomon Islands, members of the mother's family come together for a ceremony called 'causing to give birth'. The senior male relative of the family takes oil in his hand and massages the belly of the pregnant woman. By doing this he serves as a vehicle through which the power of the family ancestors can pass to the woman and her unborn child. He begins by calling on the ancestor whom the family thinks will probably be most interested in this particular birth. He then recites an incantation which will make labour and birth easier:

> Stand firm and make strong
> And give power to my hand
> Be turned the face of the little child
> Down below

(i.e. turn the child in the right direction in which to be born)

> Erect the twice breaking wave
> And send it down below

(i.e. make labour easy)

You come down onto your property
Which has been spread out
By your house of father's sisters
And your house of grandparents
That they might nurse you

(i.e. this refers to the cloth spread to receive the child at birth
and again asks the child to be born without delay)

In Java, at the first sign of labour, the midwife is called and
comes to the home of the mother. She massages the mother,
chanting the following incantation aimed at harnessing as
many positive powers as possible to ensure a quick and easy
delivery.

In the name of God the Merciful, the Compassionate
My intention is to roll out a sleeping mat
And set a loosely woven basket [the mother] upon it
Grandfather, spirit of Modjokuto
Grandmother, spirit of Modjokuto
Open the door to heaven,
Close the door to hell
The devils and other evil spirits, may they go away
The male ancestor spirits say that nothing will happen
The female ancestor spirits say that nothing will happen
Wherever you wander you may be safe
May you be safe from dangers both above and below
Wherever you wander or go, little mother
Who are about to bear a child

Towards the end of pregnancy the Ga father in Africa plays
an important role. He has to find out whether the unborn
child has any special needs or wants as only when these are
fulfilled will the child be born easily. A long white line is
drawn across the mother's abdomen and is crossed by a
second one. This causes the baby to prick up her ears and
become attentive and communicative. The medicine man
gazes into a bowl of dark liquid and listens while the child
speaks. Normally the child asks for presents of money or
eggs to be given to the 'unseen friends' (i.e. spirits) that will
accompany and help her during her journey into the world.

Money is waved over the mother's head and this, with the washing sponge, is thrown on the rubbish heap for the spirits who come and take it away and in so doing ensure that the baby is easily born.

Elsewhere in Africa the Azande father consults the oracle late in his wife's pregnancy to determine where she should give birth. The oracle tells him whether she should give birth in the hut or under a tree and who is to be the midwife and who is to sit behind the woman and help her. If all these conditions are met then the birth should not be difficult.

At the beginning of labour, or just before, is a time when offerings may be made or special prayers said to the spirits or gods who can provide most help at this time. In Haiti, at the onset of labour, sacrifices are made to Damballa and the spirits of the twins, and also to the deity which is thought to protect the unborn child. A candle will be lighted and put at the threshold of the room where the birth is to take place. A candle may also be lighted in the church before the statue of the saint who corresponds to the *vodun* deity protecting women in labour. All the different spirits, ancestors, *vodun* gods, saints and the God of the Catholic Church are invoked and offerings made; a Pater Noster and Ave Maria are said and then the following prayer addressed to whichever gods and spirits are willing to help:

> *All the gods, both of my father and my mother, as well as those of my husband. I ask that you cause me to have a good delivery, that you open the road for me. I ask the family ancestors all to come deliver me, that you open the way for me, that you do not allow evil spirits to bar my path when the time for delivery approaches. May you all, Invisible Beings, the Saints, the Dead twins, come to my aid on that day.*

It is interesting to see how in this prayer, spirits from many different sources are asked for help at this special time. Whatever the religious beliefs of the traditional midwives that I talked to in south east Asia (many were either Muslim or Christian), the incantations they used and the spiritual help that they sought often came from a much wider or older spiritual tradition. Sometimes they were rather embarrassed about this as in Malaysia, for instance, Malay Muslim mid-wives were roundly condemned for such practices by those of a more fundamentalist Islamic persuasion.

Such condemnation on the part of organized religions has a long history. In England and Europe during the fourteenth century, one reason for the Christian Church's condemnation of midwives was the charms and incantations that they used to help women in labour. Some of these undoubtedly derived from pre-Christian beliefs, but often they used Christian ones as well. Latin charms such as the following:

> O infans siue vicus. siue mortuus, exi foras, quia
> Christus te vocat ad lucem.
> (Oh infant whether living or dead, come forth because
> Christ calls you to the light.)

or the beginning of the Athenasian creed might be used, the latter being said three times over the labouring woman.

With the Reformation such 'inventions of the devil' were condemned by the Church and a midwife's oath dating from 1567 includes the promise to refrain from using sorcery or enchantments during labour. The only ritual she was allowed to use was baptism when death seemed imminent. During the seventeenth century in France, an invocation to the Virgin was used during labour and special prayers were composed for pregnant women. Rather than ensuring an easy delivery, however, they tended to stress the pain and suffering that justifiably ensued from the sinful act of conception. Despite this, such prayers continued to be used; in Ireland, holy water was sprinkled on the mother while the following was said:

> Woman, bear your child as Anne bore Mary
> As Mary bore God
> Without disfigurement or blindness
> Or lack of foot or hand.

The Christian Church has always been against the relieving of pain in labour. When chloroform was first used to prevent pain in labour in 1847 it created a furore amongst Anglican clergy who considered the technique went against the wishes of God as expressed in Genesis 3.16: 'In sorrow shalt thou bring forth your children'. For the next one hundred years this was discussed in the Church and as late as 1956, Pope Pius XII felt that he had to produce an encyclical on the subject.

Once it becomes obvious that labour has started some practical arrangements may have to be made in terms of where birth takes place and in getting the necessary helpers. Some women give birth away from their home, often in a special temporary or permanent hut built for the purpose while others give birth in their homes but often in a specially secluded room. A Batek Orang Asli mother who had recently given birth told me how a special hut had been built for her just across the river from where they were living. This was a nomadic group and the hut was built as soon as labour started, taking about half an hour to construct, after which she went to it with one of the other women in the group. In other places there may be a more permanent special place which is set apart from the other houses and to which women go when labour starts.

In some places women give birth alone although usually they are able to call for help should they need it. Amongst the Chukchee, a Siberian nomadic group, no-one is present during the birth except one old woman who, if absolutely necessary, renders assistance. The woman has her own special 'skin scraper' stone which she keeps in her clothes bag and with which she cuts the umbilical cord. Once the baby is born no stranger, and especially a man, is allowed to enter the room where the mother and baby lie in case they have evil influences clinging to them. As mentioned previously, the African Benin prefer to give birth alone as it provides the opportunity for the woman to demonstrate her courage and stoicism and thus enhance her status in the group.

Once labour starts the Aborigine woman leaves the camp where she lives with her husband. With her mother and other female relatives, one of whom acts as a midwife, she goes to the women's camp where she gives birth. Aborigine birth songs are known only to the women of the tribe and are sung to charm the pelvis and genital organs of women in the process of giving birth. They were first uttered by the female totemic ancestors, and during labour and birth the women chant these songs which tell of how the woman in labour will be able to surmount the dangers of childbirth and bear her child safely without bleeding and injurious after-effects.

The African Yoruba woman gives birth in her own home but as soon as labour starts, goes into a secluded room with a herbalist doctor, village midwife and several elders. Here she is bathed with medicinal herbs and wrapped in a light cloth. To reassure her various poems, like the following, are recited:

The goats have no midwives
The sheep have no midwives
When the goat is pregnant, she is safely delivered
When the sheep is pregnant, she is safely delivered
You, in this state of pregnancy, will be safely delivered

Once labour starts for the Cherokee woman, all children and male inmates, apart from her husband, must leave the house. Four women (there is great magical significance in this number) must come to help. They can be family, friends or neighbours, but one of them must be the midwife who knows the necessary formulae to deal with complications. She goes to all four corners of the cabin asking the baby to 'jump down' quickly; at the east and west corners the boy is asked to jump down quickly and at the north and south corners the girl. In the Sudan, the Dinka woman gives birth in a special hut and only senior women are allowed to attend although this will normally include her mother. Here the midwife is known as *geem* or 'receiver of God's gift of a child'; through carrying out this task, she becomes the spiritual mother of the child, this being remembered by the child throughout his life. Dinka women are urged, from the time labour starts, to confess any illicit sexual relations that they have had as failure to do so may lead to a difficult delivery. Usually their feelings of guilt and the fear of supernatural sanctions and threat of death encourages them to do so. If a woman dies in childbirth it is thought to be because she harboured lovers and did not confess her misdeeds.

Among the Palestinians, no men are allowed to be present at a birth, which is considered to be 'women's business'. The mother of the labouring women tries to be present together with the midwife and any other female friends and relatives who want to help. A woman who is pregnant, however, should not attend as the two unborn children may talk to each other and the birth be delayed. Menstruating women or those who have not ritually cleansed themselves after sexual intercourse are considered impure and should not be present as they may cause the labouring woman to have too long a gap between this and her next pregnancy. A childless woman who wants to conceive, however, will try to be present as watching the birth will help her have children. During labour and the pain of childbirth, heaven is thought to be open and angels go up and down so that this is a good time for everyone present to make special requests to God. Of course, if the labour is long or difficult, it is then easy to make direct requests to God for help. Given this special access to heaven the women attending the birth should act circumspectly; they should not be noisy or quarrelsome or talk about their own sufferings in childbirth.

In Thailand, at the onset of labour, the pregnant woman prays in the garden at the house of the family's protecting spirits. At the same time she prepares the ceremonial gifts for the midwife and hangs out the protective cloths in the room where she will give birth. These cloths are about 10 inches square with magical letters and drawings on them. They keep out the spirits who are attracted by the smell of blood and might come and eat the mother's internal organs. When the midwife arrives she is given gifts after which she chants, 'All good spirits in the high heavens and in the locality help and do not obstruct at this delivery. Give happiness to mother and baby.' Any helpers at the birth should also be careful in what they say. No-one should talk about a 'difficult delivery' or should use words like 'stuck', 'fastened', 'hung up' or 'stuck midway', in case they come true and the woman has a difficult birth.

In Hawaii a woman in the first stages of labour may sometimes be seized with a longing to see a certain person. This means that the baby will be very fond of that person and if possible that person is called to be present and encourage the baby to be born quickly. When the person is not available a stone is put at the door in the stead of that person and this works in the same way. Afterwards it is thrown in the sea so that it remains pure. While a Ga woman is in labour a fish net and grinding stone are placed in the doorway of her room. If any woman enters the room suffering from stomach pains or with evil influences attached to her, they are caught in the net and ground in the stone so that they cannot be transferred to the woman in labour.

In many cultures, special herbs or foods are given as soon as labour starts to strengthen and change the body so that birth happens more easily. Thai women think that the pushing or pulling 'winds' that circulate within their body and normally keep the body in a healthy balance need to be speeded up during birth. The quicker the winds circulate, the stronger will be the contractions and the expulsive forces which will break the sac of amniotic fluid and force out the water with the child. The best way of doing this is by heating the body up with 'hot' foods or 'hot' herbal concoctions which she takes as soon as labour begins. Both Minangkabau and Malay midwives told me about special herbal remedies which they gave to the woman to drink as soon as they arrived and massaged on her stomach as well. A special cake for labour used to be made in Cambridge (UK). This consisted of wholemeal flour, hemp seeds crushed with a rolling pin, crushed rhubarb root and grated dandelion root. This was mixed to a batter with milk and gin and baked in a hot oven. This would be given to the husband as well as the wife to relieve any sympathetic pains which he might experience as a result of his wife giving birth. Amongst African Americans, the clay from the nest of the dish-dauber bird was burnt and the ashes drunk. This was thought to relieve labour pains and hasten delivery.

The symbolic clearing of the way so that the child can emerge is even more important during labour and birth. A

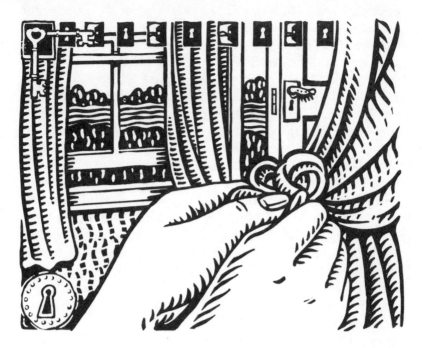

belief which is found in places all over the world is that
undoing knots and windows will ensure an easy delivery or
expedite a difficult one. In the UK, for instance, a competent
midwife would unlock all doors and loosen knots as soon as
she arrived. It was thought that malicious witches frequently
attempted to prevent delivery by tightening knots just before
or during a woman's labour and undoing them prevented
this happening. This custom took place throughout rural
Europe including Russia where the Yukaghir, in Siberia,
would loosen all knots as soon as the labour started. It was
also done in Thailand where, in addition, anyone attending
the birth would not be allowed to sit or stand in a doorway
or halfway up a flight of stairs. Sometimes this undoing of
knots would not be carried out until further on in labour or,
if there were difficulties, then everyone present might be
asked to undo knots in their clothing as well as open doors
and windows.

During the seventeenth century in France a woman in
labour liked to have by her a lighted candle and a Rose of

Jericho placed in holy water. The burning of the candle and the gradual opening of the rose corresponded to the gradual opening of her body to let the baby out. The flower had great significance for women as it was believed that 'it first blossomed at our Savour's birth, closed at the Crucifixion and opened again at Easter, whence its name the Resurrection Flower.' Thus the religious symbolism also helped women through the pain of giving birth.

Various charms were owned and used by midwives to help relieve pain and generally make delivery easier. The eagle stone has already been mentioned as a charm in seventeenth century England and once labour began it would be tied around the leg of the labouring woman. Jasper stones were sometimes used because, as well as facilitating delivery, they also helped the milk to flow after birth. The pealing of church bells was thought to aid delivery but if this could not be arranged an old bell rope tied around the mother's waist would do as well. A copy of 'Our Saviour's letter' might be hung over the bed of a labouring woman; this was an apocryphal letter said to have been written by Our Lord to Agbarus of Edessa and was thought to be particularly helpful to women in childbirth. Women in seventeenth century France used relics of saints as a means of easing pain and procuring a safe delivery. The belt or bones of St Margaret were regularly lent by convents to labouring women, but failing that her biography would be read to them instead.

There are supernatural forces and spirits which are believed to be very attracted to women in labour, often by the smell of the blood as well as by her special vulnerability. Sometimes they are ordinary evil spirits but often they only attack pregnant and labouring women, having derived from women who themselves died in childbirth. The woman is also especially sensitive to evil magic which may have been put upon her by others.

Throughout the world metal is considered to be a very efficacious charm to have around the labouring woman to neutralize these effects. In the USA it was thought to protect against witchcraft and changelings, and a very sharp axe under the bed would cut the pain in two and stop any bleeding. The husband's knife or scissors between the mattresses would ensure a quick delivery; these being considered very effective as they could be put into the shape of a cross. In the UK nails might be thrust into the wooden part of a bed with iron and other metal charms put around the room. The Malays believe that metal is very good for protecting against witches and demons that attack women in childbirth and that the metal does this by strengthening both the mother's and baby's *semangat* or spirit.

Stones have a similar effect and in the USA a stone with a hole in it was hung over the head of a woman in labour to assist in the birth and as protection against evil spirits. In Malaysia the traditional midwife puts thorny bushes under the house of the labouring woman to protect against demons of the earth that might be attracted by blood dripping through the floorboards. The Gilya in Siberia carve a wooden figure of a woman in the act of giving birth. They then sacrifice foods to it to placate the spirits who may attack the labouring woman.

WHAT FATHERS DO

In many traditional societies men are excluded from their wives at the time of birth. Where they are not, it is usually only the husband who is allowed to be present, or a ritual specialist if this is thought necessary.

Even though the father may not be present, he may nevertheless have an important part to play, the successful fulfillment of which makes him an active participant in the birth process. If his wife has any difficulties during labour or birth then his presence and participation in various rituals may be crucial in resolving problems successfully. In Ireland, a woman about to give birth wore the waistcoat or some other garment of her husband's. During the time that his wife was giving birth the husband had to undertake some symbolic work such as drawing water from a well continuously until the baby was born. This lessened the pain of childbearing for the mother by transferring it to the father. In the USA, it was believed that if a wife crossed her husband's bed at the first sign of labour then he would share in bearing the labour pains. Putting on his hat reduced pains, as would drinking water from her husband's shoes.

In some places the father actually mimics the whole process of birth and in doing so is thought to take away the labour pains from his wife to himself. The Arunta Aborigine father in Australia, as soon as labour starts, takes off all personal ornaments and whatever he has in his bags must be poured out, symbolizing the coming of the baby. If his hair is tied up or he has anything else on him which is knotted, this must be undone, all of which helps his wife to give birth more easily.

Naming the true father of the child is a way of easing the pains of labour for Yakut women (a Siberian nomadic tribe). Ga women call out the baby's father's name to give vigour to the child, waken its spirit and cause it to move a step towards being born. In cases where the woman's husband is not the child's father, the child will not move until his physical father's name is called. Thus, if birth is delayed the woman will call out the name of her lovers and when the baby's true father is called then the child will be born. This revelation may, however, have undesirable consequences for the woman in terms of divorce and it is not unknown for kindly relatives to gag the woman to ensure that no such disclosures are made.

For the Thai couple, giving birth is a joint effort in which the husband and wife are physically and emotionally united in the intense effort to deliver the child. The woman sits with her back propped up on a folded mattress, fully dressed in old clothes. The husband sits with his knees against his wife's shoulders with her head between his thighs. During intense contractions the man's thighs provide support for the woman's arms and he is able to stroke her face and hair to give emotional support. This is perhaps closest to the ideal we have in the west of the role that the father will play during birth, although in the sterile and impersonal world of the modern hospital, it may be difficult for the father to loose his inhibitions sufficiently to jump on the hospital bed to be more physically close to his wife.

In the west the role of the father has, over the last fifty years, changed dramatically. Fathers used to be pictured nervously pacing up and down hospital corridors while their wives gave birth whereas now they are more likely to be beside their wives, not just as spectators but as active participants. In America the natural childbirth movement emerged during the 1940s and with it developed the husband's role as 'labour coach'. Father participation of this kind was seen as a way of easing the wife's labour as well as strengthening the family unit. His presence at birth was not, however, easily won as, with the hospital emphasis on sterility and professional medical control in the delivery room, a non-professional outsider was not easily accommodated. Whether fathers should be present at birth became a major point of contention between medical professionals and activists in the natural childbirth movement. This led to a considerable amount of literature on expectant fatherhood during the 1960s describing the supposed benefits of father participation, which included shorter and easier deliveries, healthier mothers and babies, improvements in the quality of marital relationships and subsequent parenting. Looked at critically, most of the so-called research on which these claims were made is of dubious scientific value and there was little objective information about fathers' experience of birth. One effect, however, was that opposition to a father's presence at birth by hospitals began to fall and if not welcomed in the delivery room, he was at least tolerated there.

In the 1950s the father's attendance at birth was radical behaviour. By the 1970s it was commonplace and by the 1980s it was expected behaviour. The 'good' husband and father attended antenatal classes, coached his wife's labour and was actively involved in care of the newborn. Nowadays a father who doesn't want to be involved in this way is likely to face social disapprobation. I remember a friend of mine who felt very let down when her husband decided that he didn't want to be with her when she gave birth. Her feelings were exacerbated by the attitudes of the hospital who would

not allow anyone other than the husband to be present with
her during labour and birth. She was therefore faced with the
dilemma of either trying to persuade her reluctant husband to
be with her or of being on her own in hospital with no-one
other than hospital staff to help her.

The 'discovery' of expectant fathers during the 1970s led
to more research on their attitudes to birth, their response
to the experience and their subsequent bonding with the
newborn. Although the previous literature of the 1960s had
suggested various benefits for the whole family when fathers
participated in birth, this more rigorous research was much
more inconclusive. It does show, however, that during labour
and birth a father often feels helpless and intimidated by
hospital staff who are unsure how to treat him. He is often
asked to leave his wife if any hospital procedures are to be
carried out or if there are any complications – just the time
when his wife may feel she needs him most. A father's experience of birth is strongly affected by his own emotional reactions and the degree to which he feels able to support his
wife. It has been pointed out by one (female) researcher[5]
that the relatively passive role of protector and supporter is
counter to the masculine image of control, particularly with
respect to labour pain. Many fathers feel overwhelmed by
their wife's discomfort and the resulting feelings of helpless-
ness that it brings up within them. Research is only just
beginning to unravel some of the many influences affecting
the father's responses and experience at this time and to
break down some of the stereotypes as to what constitutes
a 'good' father.

Compared to many if not most traditional societies, this
close involvement of fathers with birth and the newborn is
a very recent phenomenon. While it may encourage fathers
to be more nurturing and thus in modern society considered
a 'good thing', it is also a reflection of the decreasing options
which many women have at this time. Whereas a woman
used to be able to turn to a network of female relatives and
friends for help and support during birth, in the small nuclear
family of modern society she may well feel that her husband
is the only person to whom she can turn. For many couples

this may well be the ideal arrangement, but for others there are often very few alternatives. Birth has become something that women share with professionals and their spouse. It is not, as in most traditional societies, something which women share with other women and which at the same time affirms their solidarity and special status within the society.

THE MOMENT OF BIRTH

I was not, unfortunately, ever able to be present at a birth with a traditional midwife, although in my travels I regularly came across mothers who had very recently given birth. In traditional societies women normally give birth in an upright position either standing, kneeling or squatting. Sometimes they hang onto a rope and I remember a Karen midwife from northern Thailand laughingly telling me that the piece of rope was the main piece of equipment which she carried from house to house. I tried it myself and it felt surprisingly comfortable and stable whereas I thought I would feel very wobbly and insecure. Yeo women (also from northern Thailand) have a rope put under their armpits and fixed to the ceiling to support them and this, too, is much more comfortable than it sounds. The Cherokee woman stands and is supported by a friend grasping her firmly under her armpits; the Maya woman sits on a small stool or squats, again supported by someone holding her from behind.

Asking about the position in which women gave birth often gave rise to much laughter on the part of my respondents as it wasn't something they thought about very much or had fixed ideas about. Many of them said it all depended on the mother and what she found most comfortable for her. Usually the midwife or her assistant would sit or stand behind the woman either to support her or to help push the baby out by massaging her stomach. Again I tried this with the Karen midwife, the whole process being carried out with sound effects much to the amusement of everyone else who had gathered around as I talked to her. One exception to this were the Malay women who usually gave birth lying on

their backs, especially, as one midwife informed me, if they
were older. I tried to find out if this was a recent phenomenon
but was told that this was how it had always been done. In
Sumatra, however, the influence of western obstetricians was
more noticeable with many midwives telling me that women
now gave birth lying on their backs instead of the traditional
kneeling on the floor and holding a rope. As always the
midwives followed the wishes of their clients, not persuading
them either way, although it was obvious that giving birth
on one's back was considered more 'modern' in comparison
to the traditional way which was considered rather old-
fashioned and 'primitive'. It is, regretfully, yet another example of how totally inappropriate methods are being exported
to third world countries. Just as we in the west are finding
the physiological and other benefits of giving birth on our
own two feet, women in third world countries are being
encouraged to lie down helplessly on their backs.

The direction in which one faces to give birth is an important consideration in some places. Carol Laderman found
that Malay midwives had a complicated system, which was
sometimes very idiosyncratic, for working this out. It
depended not only on the nature of the different directions
but also on the time and place where the birth was taking
place and had therefore to be worked out individually for
each woman as the time for birth drew near. It was important
to get the direction right so that the actual birth would be
easy and the mother and child adequately protected. Thai
women sometimes select the most advantageous direction by
looking at a hen about to lay an egg. Whichever direction
the chicken chooses the woman turns herself in the same
direction so that she gives birth as easily as the chicken lays
its egg.

In the west the majority of women give birth in hospital
which, on the face of it, is the only similarity between them
and women in traditional societies who go to a special place
to give birth. There, however, the similarity ends as, rather
than the small intimate birth hut of a traditional society,
the western woman finds herself in the large impersonal
institution of a modern hospital. Instead of being with trusted

friends and relatives whom she knows well she is, more often than not, with strangers whom she has never seen before. It is very much a lottery as to whether she will have people around her with whom she feels comfortable and in whom she has confidence that they will meet her needs.

Hospital admission methods exemplify many of the worst aspects of hospital procedures, as a detailed research project showed.[6] On coming into hospital women were often separated from their companions as a matter of course while the initial interview with hospital personnel was carried out even though this could be a time when they needed most support. The lack of privacy was felt very keenly by some women as even when they were in their own rooms, nurses and doctors felt they could walk in and out at will without knocking. Procedures ranging from the simple one of putting on a hospital gown to routine treatments such as shaving and being given an enema were often presented as if there was no choice about whether one accepted them or not. The two latter have been shown to be totally unnecessary as a preparation for birth but in some of the hospitals this was either unknown or ignored. Treating women in this way made them feel depersonalized and on a conveyor belt rather than unique individuals going through a unique experience.

During my third pregnancy, which took place while I was living in Malaysia, I saw a Malay traditional midwife regularly for massage and experienced that blend of spiritual, emotional and physical care which they provide. It would have been wonderful for this book if I could have had her attend me at birth, but Rachael had other ideas. She came three weeks early while we were on holiday and the government midwife had to be called out early one morning to help me with her precipitate arrival. It was nevertheless a wonderful and deeply satisfying experience which reminded me of Alison Campbell's[7] eloquent description of giving birth with the help of a traditional Indian midwife.

During quiet moments the midwife burned incense and sang prayers to Krishna, their protecting God, something which filled me with a feeling of solemnity at

the act of giving birth. . . . The situation provided an
understanding between us in spite of the language bar-
rier. The farmer's wife, too, filled me with confidence
and the calm solidarity of both women allayed any
fears I had. In short, they were in sympathy with me;
our communication was through mood and observance
rather than words, but it was quite satisfactory. The
atmosphere was good and generally I, and the baby
of course, were the ones to dictate the pace of the
proceedings.

The understanding and deep communication between the
labouring woman and her companions, the primacy of the
individuality of the labouring woman and the profoundness
of the moment of birth. This is the heritage we have lost and
must somehow find again if birth is to be more than just the
medical physical event it has become in the west.

PAIN IN LABOUR

When I talked to traditional midwives in south east Asia
they very rarely spontaneously mentioned anything that they
did to relieve pain. Questioning them more closely, it soon
became apparent that they thought pain was a natural part
of childbirth and they would only do anything about it if it
went on for a long time or the woman was finding it absolutely unbearable. I remember one Toraja midwife telling me
that in her opinion pain was related to fear. She said that
often when she first went to help a woman she would be
crying that the pain was too much for her, especially when
it was her first baby. Massaging her, telling her that the pain
was normal and that everything was going well was usually
sufficient to make the pains more bearable according to this
experienced midwife.

Reassurance, massage and emotional support are the
methods which traditional midwives use to relieve pain
although most of those that I talked to had some other
methods when this was insufficient during a long and difficult

labour. Usually this consisted of a local narcotic such as betel leaf given in conjunction with other things like prayers and massage, but only in extreme cases.

Women in traditional societies experience pain in labour like women everywhere, but the way that they express and deal with it takes various forms. Pain perception is related very strongly to cultural norms about how it is felt, perceived and shown and in many cultures women show their stoicism and strength by not making a noise during childbirth. Thus the meaning of pain, when it starts and ends, is reinforced by social expectations in a particular social context.

There has been little or no research on the different cultural experiences of pain in childbirth, but an interesting piece of research on dental pain[8] showed the nature of differing social expectations of pain very clearly. The sample consisted of a total of eighty-five subjects from Anglo-American, Mandarin Chinese and Scandinavian immigrants of first generation ethnicity living in Seattle, USA. About half were dentists, all of whom had been trained in their country of origin, and the rest were patients. The Chinese described the pain of tooth drilling as dull and not internal and linked it to their indigenous medical ideas of yin/yang balance. By contrast, the Anglo-Americans described the pain as sharp and intense and associated with bodily injury. As well as these differing perceptions, the two groups also had differing responses, the Chinese patients preferring externally applied agents and disdaining local anaesthetics while the Anglo-Americans had completely contrary views, preferring to have an injection. On the other hand, regardless of ethnic background, the dentists all had similar perceptions about remedies and offered everyone local anaesthesia.

The degree of pain experienced in labour will therefore depend not only on the physical stimulus but also on the emotional state of the woman and cultural expectations. In the west we tend to believe that all pain can and should be relieved by medical means, and to expect relief at low levels of suffering. This may, of course, be reinforced by hospital procedures which provide pain relief as the first line of therapy rather than as a last resort. Many woman have described how they felt under pressure to accept pain relief even when they thought they could probably have managed without it.

The issue of pain is a problematic one for hospital personnel, as was shown by a research study[9] which investigated the attitudes of 128 Swedish midwives about the measures they used to provide pain relief. Nearly two-thirds of them felt that pharmacological methods of pain relief were used too frequently and that other methods such as hot baths, relaxation techniques and massage were used too rarely. Over a half (58 per cent) thought mothers were given too little information about the risks to the baby of different sorts of analgesia and three-quarters (77 per cent) said that mothers had too little information about other methods provided. These midwives, were, however, in a quandary as they didn't want to frighten mothers as most of them would, in the end, be given drugs for pain relief.

As Michel Odent says, it is now rare for a woman to give birth entirely with her own hormones and for a baby to be born undrugged, and often more than one drug is used. When such drugs are used so widely, we should be certain of their safety but this is very difficult to do and few of the necessary clinical studies have been carried out. As far as we can tell, these drugs do not have any long-term consequences for the baby but there has been no proper research to show definitely that this is so.

A very large proportion of the midwives in the above sample (96 per cent) believe that the need for analgesics was reduced when they were present and providing emotional support for the labouring mother. It is well known that the body is capable of making its own analgesics in the form of endorphins which change the perceptions of pain, sometimes eliminating it completely. Those who have experienced various sorts of trauma say that often they feel no pain and in certain situations such as during sporting events, injuries can be completely disregarded. It is known that various sorts of stress, including that experienced during childbirth, are closely correlated with changes in the level of endorphins in the blood and thus tolerance to pain. Stress is also closely related to the imagination so that affecting the imagination with various images or with music can raise the level of endorphin secretion and thus change pain perception.

In recent years the nature of the immune system and its relationship to the mind has come under intensive scrutiny. The immune system, which includes blood cells which fight off infections as well as various chemicals in the blood such as endorphins, has been found to be closely related to the mind through the autonomic nervous system and the hypothalamus in the brain. I have already described how emotions such as anger and fright are translated into physical changes in the body, especially in terms of the changes in blood chemistry. Changes in the mind lead to changes in the body which, it has been surmised, is the main way in which shamans and traditional healers do their work. These practitioners influence the minds of their patients which in turn alter their body processes, bringing about a cure. It has been found that by creating certain images in the mind, the immune system can be strengthened and body processes altered.

This information is being used by some doctors treating chronic and incurable diseases like AIDS and cancer which may be unresponsive to biomedical therapy. Practices such as imaging and meditation have been shown to be very helpful in treating such diseases and sometimes bringing about a complete cure.[10,11] In reading about this work I have been interested to see that the doctors involved often work with a wider view of the nature of medicine than the usual narrow biomedical/physical one, although this doesn't always endear them to their more conservative colleagues.

'The pain doesn't feel so bad when there are a lot of people around to help you', was how one Malay mother explained to me how she coped with the pain of labour. The influence of the group is, in some places, extremely powerful and research suggests that this could be as much physical as entirely emotional. Substances called pheromones are introduced into the outside environment through secretions in urine and sweat. These make contact with other people through the sense of smell and in some animals have a powerful effect on the reproductive system, by affecting the other's hormonal state and readiness to mate. In humans they are thought to have effects on closely knit groups. It has been found, for instance, that groups of women living together tend to coordinate their menstrual cycles. I think that the pheromones given out by birth attendants may well have a considerable impact on the labouring woman. The chemistry of confidence that traditional midwives exude is, I am certain, very different from the chemistry of fear and doubt which is so often felt in the atmosphere of a modern hospital.

During labour and birth, which is a natural process, the primal brain or hypothalamus regulates the hormonal secretions necessary for birth to happen successfully. This is something that has to be allowed, rather than forced, to happen, and one way of doing this is to reduce the inhibitions that come from the cortex or thinking part of our brain. This can be done by providing the labouring woman with a quiet and private room with people who make her feel safe enough to surrender to her primitive instincts.

Childbirth brings a change in the state of consciousness akin, I believe, to that achieved by shamans and mystics. It is a time when a woman reaches beyond normal perceptions and may involve a vision of the universe which transcends ordinary reality. It is a time when we reach down into the very depth of our being to find the resources to give birth. Of course, in the west we are unused to moving in these realms of consciousness and we have lost our knowledge of how to support someone who is doing so.

This is not the case in traditional societies where this kind of consciousness, along with the dreaming state, is not only more a part of normal life but is also considered an important means of communication for both individuals and the group as a whole. The majority of modern doctors do not understand this and by giving women powerful analgesics too quickly, they deny them the opportunity to explore and use these dimensions and to find and use their own resources to give birth. Of course, these different sorts of consciousness can feel very uncomfortable, particularly for women who are unused to them and for whom the loss of conscious control can feel very primitive and scary. In a traditional society, of course, the birth attendants understand and know how to help a woman in this state. There is no reason why we cannot explore and learn to use these other states of consciousness more fully in the west; to invest in our own different dimensions of the mind, to become more aware and comfortable with them. If we can use the resources of our minds more fully, we can all tap our abilities to give birth, rather than investing in ever more powerful (and probably dangerous) analgesics which will divorce us even more from our own internal resources.

COPING WITH DIFFICULTIES

The traditional midwives I talked to did not expect to have to deal with many difficulties as, in their experience, most women gave birth without problems. They were all, however, supremely confident that they could deal with any complications that might arise, especially when they had the help of a guiding spirit to whom they could turn for more powerful assistance. Their confidence impressed me greatly and in fact, if too many of the women they attended had problems which they could not deal with successfully, they would not be doing the work. Women would not come to them as it would be thought that they no longer had the necessary supernatural mandate or that their practical expertise was failing.

The major physical means of dealing with a difficult delivery is massage although in some cases more drastic measures such as shaking and standing on the mother's abdomen may be used. The midwives I talked to in south east Asia all used massage extensively. If delivery was long or seemed to be delayed, massage would be used both as a means of helping the mother to cope with the pain and for turning the baby into a better position where it could be born more easily. Massage during pregnancy was something that traditional midwives were keen to undertake as they said that if the mother came to them before birth they would massage the baby into the right position for birth so that delays during birth could be avoided. They could massage a baby lying in

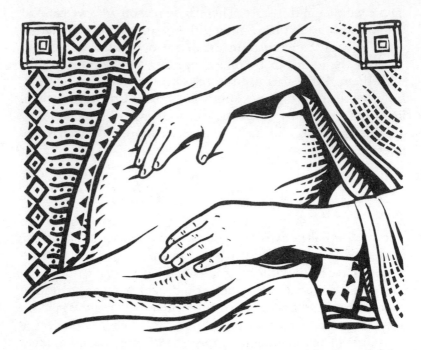

the breech position so that it would turn and be born in the normal head first way, but most would not attempt this after labour had started.

Many of the midwives I talked to had never attended a breech delivery as, compared to modern midwives, they delivered few babies so that their statistical chances of having to deal with such a delivery were very low.

The number of babies that a traditional midwife delivers depends on many factors including her age and experience, her catchment area and who else may be practising, as well as the numbers of women using other facilities like clinics and hospitals. Some women delivered several babies a month and it was almost a full time job while others only delivered a few babies each year.

Breech deliveries are not that common and may well be less common in traditional societies where the expectation is that the baby will be born head first. The other factor is that many traditional midwives turn the baby while it is in the uterus so that it will not be a breech delivery. It is of course exceptionally difficult to get hard evidence of numbers of babies born with breech deliveries from traditional societies. This is likely to remain speculative until someone manages to do some research on it over an extended period of time.

Nevertheless, all the midwives were confident that they could cope with the possibility of a breech delivery. I talked to one midwife of 75 who had just delivered her first breech baby in the previous month. She told me how she had carried it out and it sounded as if she had used techniques similar to those which I read about in modern midwifery texts, although she said that it was her guiding spirit who had instructed her how to do it. Breech deliveries were thought to be very unusual but not hazardous; such births took longer but with massage and with extra emotional support for the mother there was no reason why there should be any special difficulties.

At the same time, however, measures to enlist supernatural help will also be taken. A popular way of doing this is through the drinking of various sorts of exorcising water. In Thailand this can be made in many ways; soaking a charmed amulet in water, pouring water over the big toe of the husband, or throwing it up on the roof and catching it. Sometimes the water will be enchanted with a spell that is humorous and obscene which must be pronounced very loudly so that the woman in labour hears it. Perhaps this helps the mother to relax so that her body can give birth easily. A Malay midwife I met prayed over a glass of coconut water so that her guiding spirit was infused into it. When the labouring woman drank this the spirit was taken into her body and helped the baby to be born. In Egypt, when the birth is delayed for a long time, the husband washes his right heel and gives the water to the mother to drink. He then walks around the village seven times, not speaking to anyone. Immediately the walk is accomplished the child will be born.

In many places a difficult birth is thought to be the result of family ill feeling so that measures must be taken to deal with this if the birth is to proceed easily. Amongst the Toraja, in Indonesia, the husband will wash the back of his feet and give the water to the mother to drink. This is symbolic of washing away all ill feeling or sins that may be between them; when these are gone then the baby will be born. Among the Palestinians, if a married couple were known not to agree and the birth was difficult, the husband would wash his feet and give the water to the woman to drink, this symbolizing that they forgave each other. The Minangkabau are a matrilineal culture where descent is traced through the mother rather than the father. A Minangkabau midwife told me that if there were difficulties during birth she would ask the woman's mother to come. The labouring woman would ask her forgiveness and when it had been given, birth usually followed very quickly. If this was not effective other members of the family would be brought in, including the husband, but she said that in her experience this was rarely necessary.

If labour is prolonged amongst the Siberian Yukaghir, the midwife asks the woman, 'Who is the cause of this pregnancy?'. The husband then has to place his arm across his wife's abdomen after which the baby will be born. A researcher described an interesting case where quite a few people knew that the husband was not the biological father of the child. Nevertheless, when the midwife asked this question the woman named her husband, who then placed his arm on her stomach even though, he too, knew that he was not the biological father. By doing this, however, he accepted this fact and everyone felt the woman had spoken the truth when she said he was the father as he had accepted her and the child and would be the one to bring the child up. Apparently, the baby was born very quickly after this had happened.

A difficult delivery can also be caused by an evil spirit entering the woman. This can come about from a failure of the woman or her husband to observe certain taboos, or the ill will of the unborn child. In this situation the presence of the husband is necessary 'to loosen that which is fastened' even though during a normal delivery he will not be present.

Labouring women are, of course, very vulnerable to and easily affected by evil spirits. If a Ga woman is having difficulties the first resort will be to get a broom and give her a good sweeping to clear away evil influences. For the Palestinians, a difficult birth means that God is sparing of mercy towards the woman or that the evil eye might be upon her. A rosary from Mecca is put around her neck and she inhales the smoke from a lighted rag to destroy the evil eye. In Hawaii a complicated delivery might be the result of offending a family god so prayers and offerings are made to the ancestors.

Methods to induce the baby out of the womb are used by the Cherokee. In a long labour the mother's vagina will be washed with a concoction of herbs that 'scare' the child. Formulae may also be recited enticing the child to hurry up, as an ugly granny or the terrible-looking *flint* (a mythical being) is said to be approaching. Bribery may also be resorted to, with the child being lured out by promises of playthings, a spear for a boy and a sieve or loom for a girl, the child being given a name to increase the efficiency of this. The gypsies also call on the baby, dropping an egg between the legs of the labouring woman and chanting:

> *The egg, the little egg is round*
> *All is round*
> *Little child, come in health*
> *God, God is calling you.*

The husband plays an important part if an Aborigine woman is having a difficult delivery. She will, of course, be far away from her husband in the special women's camp, but if there are problems the husband will first take off all his personal adornments and empty his bag onto the ground. If this fails to work he will take some hair off his head which will be taken to the women's camp by a man who has a religious relationship to him. Here the man will tie the hair around the woman tightly under her breasts. If this does not work, the husband must go to the women's camp himself and walk up and down outside to induce the unborn child to follow him which, it is said, the baby rarely fails to do.

In Sarawak, when birth is delayed, two medicine men are called. One goes inside the room with the mother and the other stands outside on the veranda of the house. The one inside puts a loop of cloth around the woman while the one outside puts a similar loop of cloth around himself in which a stone is slung. Then follows a long incantation sung by the man outside during which the man inside uses all his psychic power to force the child downwards to compel delivery. When finished the cloth is tied tightly around the mother to prevent the child moving up. The one inside shouts to his companion who moves the stone downwards on his own body. This proceeds until the baby is either born or until everyone becomes convinced of the fruitlessness of these efforts.

If these normal methods fail then the midwife calls on a more powerful person to divine what the problem is and what further measures need to be taken. In a complicated delivery amongst the Dinka, once the woman's sexual morality is beyond doubt, a diviner is called in to reveal the causes of the difficulty. Contravening the rights of deities or ancestors, concealing a crime or moral wrong, and leaving wrongs amongst others uncorrected are the most common reasons. Suitable rites to make atonement are recommended, after which the baby should be born. In Haiti a priest divines whether or not the deities who have been propitiated are satisfied. If the answer is negative then minor offerings might be made immediately and the promise made for future larger offerings. Suitable rituals are enacted if the cause is displaced ancestors or because evil magic is being used against the woman.

If it is thought that evil spirits are causing difficulties by having entered the woman then an exorcist may be called in to get rid of them. In Sri Lanka the *edura* or exorcist administers holy water to the woman and carries out other ceremonies aimed at making the spirits leave the mother. When this happens to a Lahu woman in northern Thailand, a bamboo table is made. The priest or headman then uses his hands to take the spirit out of the woman and puts it into the bamboo table. This is then taken, with offerings, out into the jungle from where the spirit originated in the first place and where it can do no more harm. The Orang Asli *bomoh* in Malaysia whispers to the spirits, especially the good ones, to come and help the mother and to banish evil influences.

During an awkward delivery in Hawaii, someone is sent to gather leaves from the morning glory plant on the beach. The number of leaves varies but must always be in units of four. Half are picked with the right hand while addressing a prayer to Ku, the god of medicine, and half with the left hand addressing Hina, the goddess of medicine. The ones gathered in the right hand are eaten by the mother while those gathered in the left are crushed and rubbed on her abdomen. The Apache from America believed that a difficult delivery was a supernatural punishment for a woman who was mean and wicked. If external pressure on the abdomen and various herbal concoctions failed to have any effect, then the horse ceremony would be undertaken as horses give birth easily. If this, too, failed then the bowstring ceremony was enacted in case the baby was being kept back by the umbilical cord around its neck.

Sometimes the wider context and the nature of the universe is invoked. In Malaysia the midwife instructs the husband to step over his wife's supine body three times, this graphically illustrating which sex is on top. The woman may have been unfaithful and/or strayed from her prescribed feminine role by not being passive and submissive enough. By acting out the different roles of man and woman in this way, order and harmony as they should exist in the universe are re-established and the baby can be born. If the woman is suspected of infidelity she may be asked to drink water in which her husband's penis has been dipped, again establishing her husband's dominance.

In some places, the shaman chants a myth about birth to the labouring woman. One of the most well-known of these is the chant of the Cuna in South American. This is a long, ballad-like song which describes how men and women are created. Levi Strauss has used a psychoanalytic approach to determine how such chants can be translated into therapeutic efficiency. He proposed that it helped the mother by putting her sufferings in a wider context and that it made her feel better by helping her to see that her sufferings would result in the successful delivery of her baby. Carol Laderman found a similar kind of chant amongst the Malays but didn't think that it worked in quite the same way. One woman who had had this treatment from a *bomoh* said that she was unaware of the words that were being said and in any case, Carol Laderman felt that there were many allusions in the chant that only a *bomoh* could possibly understand.

In many cultures, if all these things fail and the mother dies in childbirth, then it is usually seen as a fault with the mother rather than a failure of the midwife. If a Ga woman dies in labour it means that she has murdered the child and special rites must be performed by officials of the goddess of birth and death. If a Batak mother dies in childbirth she is considered to have committed some crime against her *tondi* or spirit. The *tondi* no longer wished to stay near her body so the mother died. Women who die in this way are considered dishonourable and are not given a proper burial but are thrown under the house and burnt. In Thailand, if either the mother or baby dies this shows that they were not in a good karmic state and that they had not sufficient merit for the baby to want to stay with that family. In the Philippines, however, it is believed that for forty-four days after birth, the gate of heaven is open so that if a mother dies during that time she is assured of a place there.

Since the development of modern obstetrics in the last fifty years the number of women dying in childbirth and the number of babies who die soon after birth has been greatly reduced. Modern obstetricians are quick to take the credit for this and it does seem that these reduced figures go hand in hand with the growth of antenatal care and greater hospitalization of birth. On closer inspection, however, these benefits for mother and child can be explained by other things. Better nutrition, sanitation and housing brought about changes in maternal and neonatal mortality before the wholesale introduction of antenatal care. It is not at all clear that hospitalization is actually safer or brings about any other benefits for mothers and their children. The countries with the lowest rates of maternal and neonatal deaths have a very low rate of hospital births.

Modern obstetrics is, however, very good at dealing with serious problems and there are many mothers who owe their lives or the lives of their babies to the benefits of skilled obstetric care. It has also, of course, enabled a few women to give birth to children who would otherwise never have been able to do so. This group is, however, very small as the vast majority of mothers can give birth naturally with no problems. Figures vary, but it has been estimated that only 5–15 per cent of mothers actually need obstetric intervention of some kind in order to give birth. Unfortunately, modern obstetrics has become problem-focused, some would say problem-obsessed given that even a normal pregnancy is treated as a medical condition which has to be managed by medical professionals who assume that, with obstetric intervention, all births are safer.

Marjorie Tew,[12] who has carried out a careful statistical analysis of the effects of obstetric interventions, shows that the reverse is true. In the years between 1969 and 1981 in the UK, a large percentage of births took place in hospital with obstetric management of childbirth and consequent routine interventions of various kinds. There was a concomitant decrease in the perinatal mortality rate (the number of babies who die within a week of birth) and it was assumed that the former caused the latter although no valid analysis of data was taken to justify this assumption. Marjorie Tew carried out such an analysis and found that in the years when the percentage of hospital births increased, the perinatal mortality rate decreased least and vice versa. In other words, although the perinatal mortality rate continued to decrease overall, it decreased less when the percentage of hospital births rose and more when the percentage of hospital births was stationary or fell.

While this may be true for normal births, what about those women at risk of obstetric complications? Evidence from the survey of British Births 1970 was analyzed in which a large sample of women were allocated a score depending on the extent to which it was thought they were at risk of various complications. This was based on a number of factors such as whether they had an pre-existing problems like diabetes or epilepsy, as well as whether they developed high blood pressure or toxaemia during pregnancy or were expecting a breech birth. As might be expected, those with higher 'at risk' scores were more likely to give birth in hospital, but at every risk level there was a higher perinatal mortality rate for those giving birth in hospital than for those who gave birth elsewhere. What was most disturbing was that for those at low and medium risk the difference between hospital and birth elsewhere was greatest. Giving birth in hospital therefore increased the risk that the baby would die, especially for those women who were only at low or medium risk to start off with.

Further support for the value of community care by midwives was demonstrated in research[13] in Holland where 1692 mothers in Gronigen were interviewed three weeks after the birth of their babies. Some 12 per cent of these mothers had to be closely supervised by an obstetrician and to give birth in hospital because of medical problems. The rest, however, were normal healthy women who chose where and how they gave birth, with 23.4 per cent giving birth at home, 32.3 per cent going to hospital and staying 24 hours, and the remaining 32.6 per cent going to hospital and staying seven days. Their choice of place in which to give birth determined whether they were likely to have problems or not. Only 15.6 per cent of women booked for a home delivery were referred to an obstetrician during delivery compared with 25.3 per cent of women booked for a hospital birth. Women who opted for a home confinement had significantly fewer complications during pregnancy, delivery and after than those opting for birth in hospital, where more babies died than when birth took place at home. This study provides yet more evidence that for normal healthy women, giving birth in hospital is itself a cause of problems.

Despite the results of these studies a woman wanting to give birth at home is likely to face many difficulties, not the least of which are the experts' assurances that a hospital delivery is safer. As Mary Cronk and Caroline Flint explain in their book *Community Midwifery*,[14]

It concerns us that when we book a woman for a home birth we are expected to list to her all the dangers of having a baby at home so that we are sure that the decision is a result of informed choice. However, when a woman books into a hospital for a hospital birth is she ever given a list of the dangers of hospital birth? Or even the dangers of a hospital birth in that particular unit? Imagine her being told: 'We think we ought to tell you that in this unit we have a particularly resistant staphylococcus which crops up from time to time, and we have a consultant obstetrician whose caesarian rate is twice the national average and you are booked under him. Also the epidural team is having problems getting its quota of epidurals practised by their learners, so that every woman here is under great pressure to have an epidural and our percentage is running at 65% of having epidurals this month.' It makes you think.

It does indeed.

In the environment of modern obstetrical care the support and confidence in themselves that women need to give birth successfully is destroyed. They find it harder and harder to give birth naturally and the need for medical intervention is increased. A vicious cycle has been set up in which antenatal and natal care is, while helping a few women with problems, at the same time causing more problems and increased medical intervention for everyone else. This is very good for doctors wanting to make more money and expand obstetric services but does not serve the needs of the majority of women who want a normal birth.

CHAPTER FOUR

AFTER BIRTH

DELIVERING THE PLACENTA AND CUTTING THE CORD

A baby may have been safely delivered, but in many cultures will not be considered fully born until the placenta has also arrived. Often the umbilical cord cannot be cut or the baby picked up (even though it may seem to be in distress) until this has happened. In many parts of South America it is thought that if the cord is cut there is nothing to pull the placenta downwards and it will rise up in the mother's body and choke her. Few of the midwives I talked to in south east Asia had experienced any problems with the delivery of the placenta although most were aware of the problems which might occur if it did not appear reasonably soon after birth. Generally, they either just waited for it to appear or massaged the mother's stomach to help it on its way. The placenta was usually delivered within twenty minutes of the baby's arrival although exceptionally it could take up to two hours; only after that period of time would the midwife feel that perhaps more active measures were necessary to ensure that it was delivered successfully.

In Malaysia, an Indian midwife told me that if the placenta did not appear after a reasonable time she would stuff the mother's hair in her mouth. This would most likely induce vomitting which always had the effect of expelling the placenta. The Cherokee use a similar method although here vomiting is induced with a mixture of herbs. African Americans used to get the woman to blow into her fist or a bottle, or if this didn't work to snuff up red pepper through a goose quill. The subsequent sneezing and coughing reflex was usually sufficient to expel the placenta. The mother might also be made to stand or sit over a bucket of hot coals on which feathers would be burned until she was thoroughly smoked. In medieval Germany a retained placenta was treated by first cutting a cross into the mother's back with a knife. This was then plunged into the earth with a suitable Christian charm which exorcised the worms in the womb that were withholding the placenta.

Birth can be long and difficult because of the effects of evil spirits or magic and this can also be an important factor in the ease with which the placenta is delivered. Working as a researcher amongst the Tzeltal Indians in Mexico, Florence Gerdel[1] came across a case of this nature. A woman had given birth to a baby girl but after several hours the placenta still hadn't arrived and her family were beginning to fear for both her and the baby's safety. Her abdomen felt hard and hot and a rope had been tied around her waist in an effort to stop the placenta from rising any further in her body. A witch doctor was called in an attempt to determine who had cast a curse upon the mother. After feeling the pulses in both her wrists and consulting with the woman's family he revealed who had put a curse upon the woman. She confessed that this had in fact happened; the offending man was also a witch doctor and had, during her pregnancy, accused her of stealing. Following this confession one of the men lifted her up while three women pushed down on her uterus until the intact placenta suddenly appeared. With great relief the cord was then cut and other ceremonies for the newborn undertaken.

Everywhere I went in south east Asia I asked what was done about excessive bleeding after birth. Although most women seemed aware of the possibility and dangers of this happening, I was assured that this was another one of those things which was quite rare. By far the most common method was to use massage, maybe in conjunction with various herbs, these sometimes being given as a preventative measure. A Karen midwife told me that she used a special root which she dried and made into a tea which the woman then took for a few days. At the same time she needed to make sure that she sat near the fire and rested and that if she did this the bleeding would almost certainly stop. If it did not, the spirits would be asked to help, these being bribed with the sacrifice of a pig if the bleeding stopped in a short time but only a chicken if it continued for two days or more.

African Americans used to stop post-partum bleeding by applying cobwebs and soot. This would be put onto a dark cloth as a white cloth would make the blood flow too much, and then placed on the vulva. Another remedy was to heat a piece of alum with sugar and to sprinkle it on absorbent cotton. This would then be pushed into the vulva to the womb with the third finger of the right hand. The bleeding would stop more quickly if the mother was also given some cold tea made from bark taken from the north side of a cherry tree. It was also thought efficacious if the husband took off his shirt and bound it around the wife's abdomen.

Bleeding after delivery is not, however, necessarily seen as a problem. The blood that comes out after delivery is thought by many cultures to be especially dirty as it is the collection of menstrual blood which has been inside the body since the cessation of menses at the beginning of pregnancy. A Toraja midwife from Sulawesi in Indonesia told me how important it was that all this blood was completely expelled. In her opinion it was better to bleed a bit too much than not enough, as retention of this blood could lead to long-term health problems.

In some places there is considerable ritual over the cutting of the umbilical cord and the person who does this is especially chosen for this important job. In south east Asia, I found tremendous variations in where the cord is cut and the length of cord that is left hanging on the baby. The Malay midwife measures a finger's length while the Yeo midwife measures down to the baby's knee. In Mexico a hand's breadth is measured while the Cherokee measure to the baby's shoulder. The cord may be knotted before it is cut or it may be tied in one or more places, either with plant fibre or nowadays more often with cotton.

Various implements are used to cut the cord. In south east Asia a piece of bamboo may be used, cut either from a bush growing nearby or from the bamboo used to build the house or the fireplace. Sometimes a slice of turmeric root will be placed under the cord as it is being cut or a special leaf will be used for that purpose. In Mexico, the cord is cut with a sharp knife after which it is cauterized with three burning sticks taken from the fire and then a cotton dressing is firmly tied onto it. In India, the leatherworkers traditionally carry out this task, their sharp knives being prized for this purpose. All too often, however, the cord is cut with anything which comes to hand, like a trowel or a scythe which could infect the baby.

A doctor[2] who carried out research on this subject in India found that such traditional methods were not necessarily bad. He compared rates of neonatal tetanus in babies where umbilical cords had been cut with leatherworkers' knives, the scissors of western-trained midwives, and other implements such as trowels or scythes. Unexpectedly, the lowest rate of infection were found amongst those babies where leatherworkers' tools had been used, suggesting that the constant sharpening and cleaning of the tools make them a good instrument for the job. As far as I know, similar research has not been carried out on other indigenous methods but they are not necessarily unhygienic and a cause of infection. Bamboo has some natural antiseptic properties, as does turmeric and of course these items are easily obtainable and disposable. Similarly, cauterizing the cord must have some antiseptic effects and help prevent infection.

When western-type pregnancy care is introduced into third world countries, often these traditional methods of dealing with the umbilical cord are condemned. In Malaysia, for instance, cutting the cord can only be carried out by government-trained midwives using 'proper' instruments and traditional midwives must call them in to carry out this task. Thus, their traditional knowledge and skills are denigrated and the power of the government-sponsored services is established. Teaching traditional midwives to use 'modern' methods is not necessarily a good idea either, as they may not have the resources for proper sterilization. It takes 200 grams of firewood to boil a litre of water and in places where wood is scarce, this represents a considerable amount of time and effort on the part of the person, usually the woman, who is responsible for finding it.

What the placenta and umbilical cord look like can be important indicators of the future success of the child or his/her occupation. The Maya midwife in South America looks for signs on the babies she delivers to see if any of them have a supernatural mandate for being either a midwife or other spiritual practitioner. A piece of the amniotic sac on the baby's head or what looks like a sack over the shoulder both have supernatural significance. Cauls are considered significant in many parts of the world. In England they used to be thought to protect from drowning so that if a baby had a caul on its head this would be carefully dried and might be sold by the midwife to sailors for some considerable sum. There was also a belief that the person so born would never die by drowning. In addition it was thought to bestow the gift of oratory and as a result was also in demand by lawyers. Amongst the Ozark in the USA, if a child was born with a caul it was carefully dried and given to the child when it was mature, otherwise the child might be condemned to a life of perpetual misfortune. If the caul fell into the hands of an enemy the child would be in that person's power for as long as he or she had the caul.

The delivery of the placenta, which in the west is known as the third stage of labour, is usually a very hurried affair and is seen as having little or no significance for the mother. The main aim of this part of labour is to expel the placenta as quickly as possible to prevent bleeding and other complications, and to this end, until recently, most third stages were 'actively managed' even if the rest of the labour had been allowed to progress naturally.

Cutting of the cord as soon as the baby was born was first carried out during the seventeenth century, presumably so that the baby could be moved more easily and quickly from the mother. This action deprives the baby of the blood remaining in the placenta but does not affect the process by which the placenta separates from the uterus. What does happen, however, is that as the placenta contracts and is squeezed by the uterus, the remaining blood in it is squeezed out of the cut end of the cord. This makes a dreadful mess and as it was about this time that women started lying down in bed to give birth, rather than using a birthing stool, the linen was soiled.

So, soon after the early cutting of the cord was introduced, cord clamping was also used to stop the bedlinen getting dirty. This, unlike early cutting of the cord, *does* interfere with placental separation. Since the blood from the placenta cannot escape, a counter-resistance is set up, making it impossible for the placenta to become compressed and compact. This in turn makes it difficult for the uterus to contract properly and thus separation of the placenta from the uterus is slowed down. The body's response to this is to form a blood clot behind the placenta with the consequence that the mother loses more blood. Her cervical muscles may begin to retract and this, combined with the more bulky placenta, makes it more difficult, if not impossible, to expel the placenta.

Research in South Africa[3] showed that cord clamping led to a doubling of blood loss in the mother, a much higher incidence of manual removal of the placenta and a generally longer time for the placenta to be delivered.

Cutting the cord so quickly, before the baby is fully born and breathing, is thought by primal therapists to have very significant effects upon the baby's subsequent emotional and psychological development. Deprived of oxygen at the crucial moment of birth, the baby must struggle to breathe and it is this struggle and often panic experienced by the baby in this situation which these therapists believe has such far-reaching effects. This is, of course, exacerbated by the atmosphere in the delivery room where, because the baby is deprived of this auxiliary supply of oxygen through the placenta, oxygen may be given to him as a matter of course to ensure immediate breathing. A high degree of tension thus attends the moment of birth as well as interrupting the natural sequence of events by which mother and baby get to know each other.

The blood from the placenta also acts as a 'volume main-
tenance system' for the baby in that as he starts to breathe,
sufficient blood is delivered to him for his new breathing
system. When the cord is clamped early this blood is not
available and may lead to the newborn having breathing
difficulties as, without this extra blood, the necessary lung
expansion may not take place. There is evidence that the
cord will go on pulsating and providing the baby with oxygen
until he can breathe for himself. If the baby is having difficulty with breathing this support can continue for quite an
extended period of time. Of course, some babies will need
to be helped with their breathing, but to cut the cord so early
and take away this auxiliary oxygen supply for no good
reason seems unnecessarily interventionist.

Early clamping and cutting the cord interfered with the
natural separating of the placenta from the uterus and not
surprisingly, with the introduction of this practice, there was
an increased incidence of retained placenta. Doctors then
advocated pulling on the cord so that the placenta could be
pulled out before the cervix closed. This, however, had certain drawbacks: the cord might break, the placenta might be
pulled out before it separated properly, leaving a portion of
it behind, and there was always the possibility of inverting
the uterus. These factors all led to an increase in the incidence
of post-partum haemorrhage and infection, so that further
intervention with anaesthetics was necessary to manually
remove the placenta or otherwise deal with difficulties.

During the 1920s post-partum bleeding was a common
problem and accounted for 22 per cent of maternal deaths
in the UK at that time. In the 1930s the drug ergometrine was
discovered and it was found that, by giving it intravenously
immediately after birth, bleeding could be controlled. This
was hailed as a major breakthrough and maternal deaths
from this cause fell steadily until the 1940s, although it is
not clear whether this was due to the drug or the improved
nutritional and health status of the mothers. As the drug
became more readily available, it was used more widely even
though this led to an increased incidence of retained placenta

because the drug sometimes made the uterus contract onto it instead of expelling it.

An alternative drug, syntometrine, was developed in the 1960s and once this was introduced, the practice of actively managing the third stage quickly spread. Very few questioned the wisdom of giving the drug as a routine prophylactic and discussion tended to revolve around which drug was best, how to give it and the best way of delivering the placenta. Midwives were thus taught to actively manage the third stage by injecting the drug as the baby was born, clamping and cutting the cord as quickly as possible, and then delivering the placenta by pulling on the cord.

Undoubtedly, many lives have been saved by this drug, but it does not therefore follow that it is a good thing to give it to all women. Like so many things in modern obstetrics, this form of management was introduced without proper testing, although the possible problems that it could cause were known.

A research project[4] carried out in Ireland by Cecily Begley compared this type of active management with what she called 'physiological management' – allowing the placenta to be expelled without outside interference. All 1429 women in the trial were considered at low risk of post-partum haemorrhage and were randomly assigned to the two different forms of management of the third stage. Those who had an actively managed third stage were statistically more likely to have a manual removal of the placenta and in this group there was an increased likelihood of secondary post-partum bleeding. They were also more likely to suffer from nausea, vomiting, severe afterbirth pains and high blood pressure. The incidence of blood loss greater than 500ml and a post-natal haemoglobin of 10 grams/100 (indicating anaemia) were greater in the physiologically managed group, but there was no difference in the need for a blood transfusion.

The conclusions were that the routine use of ergometrine and the consequent active management of the third stage of labour for those at low risk of haemorrhage was not necessary and had many adverse effects. It was true that those who were not actively managed did bleed more but the amount lost was no more than that withdrawn at a routine blood donation. This loss should not cause problems for normal healthy women and in fact, the majority of women did not suffer any further consequences. Such a blood loss usually counts as a post-partum haemorrhage but perhaps, in the light of these findings, this should be reviewed.

Cecily Begley thinks that other physiological methods should be investigated, in particular whether less use of episiotomy and more suckling of the baby immediately after birth would diminish even this blood loss. Again, it seems, interfering with the natural processes of birth causes more problems for normal women than letting nature take its course.

DEALING WITH THE PLACENTA

To most people in the west the placenta is merely a piece of tissue with no particulary virtues once the baby has been born. The wonderful way in which it has nurtured the baby for the nine months of its growth inside the mother is rarely acknowledged and most women don't even see it. Placentas are disposed of either as a piece of waste or they are sent to drug companies so that the hormones contained within them can be extracted. To people in traditional societies, the placenta is much more than that and its proper disposal, which is often carried out by the father, is essential to the child's future growth and development.

In Nigeria, the Yoruba believe that the child is not only physically but supernaturally attached to the placenta and there is considerable significance in the way it is disposed of. It can be put in a pot and buried outside the father's house so that in later life the child will look back to it and not neglect the family. Sometimes it is buried near a river so that when it is covered with water during the rainy season it will protect the child from fevers. The Malays call the placenta the baby's 'little brother' which develops during the second month inside the womb. As the baby grows, it grows away from its sibling and hence develops the umbilical cord. When the baby is born this little brother is buried somewhere near the house. The Minangkabau believe that if you want the child to stay near home, you should bury the placenta under the front step of the house; then however much the child subsequently travels, they will always return home. If you want the child to travel and make a fortune (which is a great Minangkabau tradition), you should bury the placenta away from the house or throw it in the river.

The placenta can be important for the newborn's future health. The Karen in northern Thailand put the placenta and cord in a bamboo water pipe (often now a plastic bottle) and either bury it by a tree or tie it to the branches. The placenta contains one of the baby's souls so if the baby subsequently becomes ill one can ask the spirits to contact the soul in the placenta and ask the baby's soul to come back. It is also thought that by putting it in a water pot, the baby's heart will remain cool and so she will not suffer from fevers.

The Lahu, also from northern Thailand, put the placenta and cord in a bamboo water pot and bury it under the house. According to one mother, this was the agreement they had with the spirits and if it was not done then the baby might become ill. The Batek Orang Asli also bury the placenta but before they do this they take a piece of the cord, dry it and then tie it around the baby's neck for protection from the spirits that cause illness. A little hair is also shaved off the head and put in a bag tied around the neck for the same reason.

Sometimes there is a more elaborate ritual, such as that performed by the Akkha in northern Thailand. Immediately after the birth, the husband kills a chicken which he gives to the mother to eat. He then mixes the chicken soup with the placenta and cord and takes it to a pole outside the house to which the ancestors are thought to be attached. He digs a hole, buries the placenta and puts a stick to mark the position. For seven days, he pours boiling water over the place where he has buried it, after which he throws the stick away. The person who told me about this said that this ritual ensured that the baby's cord would drop off very quickly and without problems.

In Guatemala, the umbilical cord of the girl is put under a hearthstone so that she stays at home and helps her mother when she grows up. The cord of a boy is hung up in the granary so that he works well and productively in the field. When the Karen man goes out to bury the placenta, he will cut a stick from a bush or tree on his way back. If the child is a girl the stick symbolizes her weaving stick whereas if it is a boy it symbolizes his gun, ensuring that they will be good at their respective tasks when they grow up. I was told by a Batak midwife from Sumatra that if you buried the placenta with a little kerosene this stopped the baby crying at nights. In Tana Toraja, if a woman has had several children who have died she hangs the placenta of her latest baby on a palm tree as this stops the baby dying, although the midwife I spoke to couldn't tell me why this was so.

The Cherokee father must take the placenta and cross two mounain ridges before burying it with a special incantation which says that it will be two years before the placenta sees another child. If he would like another child after only one year he crosses only one mountain ridge. He has to be very careful that no-one sees him, as an enemy would be able to dig the placenta up and rebury it very deeply so that the couple did not have any more children, or throw the placenta away so that the couple have another baby before they want to.

PROTECTING THE MOTHER AND NEWBORN BABY

Anyone who has given birth knows the delight of those first few hours after birth. An undrugged baby is particularly alert at this time so it can be a wonderful period of communication, of getting to know each other and starting to breast-feed. This, of course, is known as 'bonding' but I've never read anything in the medical literature which even approaches a description of the sheer delight that it can be for both mother and baby.

For the woman in a traditional society this period extends much further than the few hours or so (sometimes a few minutes only) that one normally gets in the hurried atmosphere of a modern hospital. After giving birth, both mother and baby are thought to be at special risk, the mother because of all her exertions and the subsequent weakening of her body, and the baby because of the sudden change in environment and possibility that his or her soul is not yet firmly established in the body. For this reason there are often rituals that have to be undertaken as well as a period of exclusion for the mother. This may or may not be combined with notions of purification and may also include various food taboos which she must observe to both restore her health and make sure that her milk supply is good.

Immediately the Ga baby is born, the father's sister is sent to the medium to consult the oracle and find out whether the child has any special wishes that need to be fulfilled, from which family it came and whether any special rites are required. Until she returns, the mother must sit with the unwashed baby in her arms. On the sister's return the baby's wishes, as described by the medium, must be fulfilled and any necessary ritual undertaken. After this both the baby and its parents are bathed and blessed together by the priest. The baby is kept 'like an egg' indoors for seven days; if after this time the baby is still alive and healthy, he or she is said to have survived the seven dangers and to be worthy of being called a person.

In Korea, the inner room where the mother has given birth becomes a sacred space which shelters the mother and baby from potentially dangerous forces outside. The family must guard the ritual cleanliness of the room so that the Birth Grandmother is not offended. After the birth, this goddess must be greeted with elaborate gifts and for three days after the birth, rice and soup are offered to her. At the same time the mother prays to her 'to make the milk flow' and consumes special food to ensure a good lactation. Only members of the household are allowed to enter the room after birth.

New babies are very vulnerable and have to be protected both physically and from malevolent spirits and other forces.

In Egypt after a Christian gives birth, relatives mix wheat flour with water to make a dough. Crosses are made out of this mixture and stuck to the walls of the room occupied by the mother and child, the greatest number being put close to where the child lies. Christian baptism is a very important rite for gypsies as until this is performed, the child is unclean and doesn't exist properly as a person. Muslims have special prayers which are said soon after the birth of the child either by the father, grandfather or grandmother, so that the child is protected.

In Sarawak, if it rains when the sun is shining, this is thought to be very injurious to health and newborn babies have to be especially protected. Special leaves are burnt, the smoke from which drives away any spirits hovering nearby. In Hawaii, the clothes used during childbirth have to be very carefully guarded as they could be used for evil magic. Only the mother herself or a trusted family member is allowed to see them or to wash them.

In Ireland it used to be feared that fairies always tried to take away newly born children and talismans were given to the mother to stop this happening. For two days after birth in an Akkha village (in northern Thailand), the whole family must stay in the village in case evil spirits from the jungle and other places outside the village cling onto them and affect the baby. When I visited a very new mother in an Akkha village, I didn't realize their feelings about outsiders and touched the baby. The mother was very concerned that I might have inadvertently brought evil spirits with me so just to make sure that I neutralized all possible evil effects, I tied a piece of white cotton around the baby's wrist. I then gave the baby a silver coin which he grasped, showing that everything was probably all right.

The winnowing ceremony is carried out by Thai parents during the first three days of the child's life. The child is taken and gently dropped onto a winnowing basket while all the family stand around. As this is being done one of the parents has to shout 'mine' and the first one to do so 'owns' the child. If another member of the family does this he or she becomes like a godparent to the child. It is said that, as

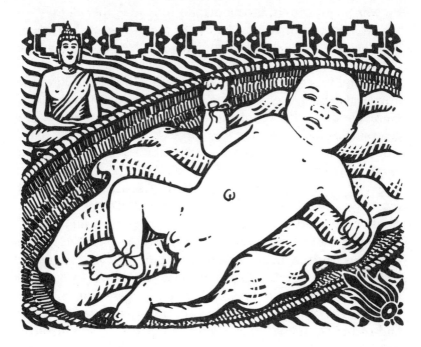

the baby is dropped on the basket, the shock 'makes him forget life as a spirit' and therefore anchors him more firmly in his body. When someone shouts 'mine', this also cuts his connection with the spirit world and he becomes fully human.

Holy thread is then tied at the wrists and ankles of the child, tying the soul to the body, providing it with a lifelong home and giving the child membership of the family. Whoever announced responsibility for the child's care, usually the mother, deserved reciprocal care from the child in her old age. Various items are put on the basket with the child, these being chosen according to the characteristics which the parents want imparted to the child. Waywardness is very much feared so magic might also be invoked to keep the child close to home. A blessing will be said invoking immovable things – a post outside the house, a cat that doesn't leave home – so that the child will absorb these characteristics and not leave home easily.

Naming the child is often a ritual with special significance.

In some cultures it is important to name the child very quickly after birth so that he or she is not named and taken by other spirits. The Akkha midwife does this as soon as the baby appears, the name being chosen according to how many other children there are in the family. In some cultures, however, names are not given until the child is much older. Names may be given informally but more often there is a ceremony such as that carried out by the Minangkabau, where the name is given when the baby is first taken down to the river to be bathed. This is a family occasion also attended by the religious leader who snips a few hairs off the baby's head and names him or her. There is usually a small party and meal for all members of the family and especially for the midwife who attended the birth.

Sometimes the name is so important that it cannot be chosen by the family alone but must be divined by various means with the help of supernatural forces. The Siberian Chukchee mother holds a divinatory object in front of her and recites the names of the family ancestors. At the mention of the correct name the object loses its balance. She may also name the child after the first object she comes across after giving birth, or as a result of dreams. If the baby does not thrive then the name may be changed by a shaman. In India, after the birth of a baby Hindus go to the temple and ask the priest for a horoscope. Amongst other things, this shows what letters and sounds the name should contain if the child is to keep healthy and be lucky.

The Chinese also set great store by names, these being chosen for their associations with the characteristics of objects or animals. If it seems that the child is unlucky or has a lot of ill health, a medium will be called in to decide how the name should be changed to change the person's circumstances. Sometimes babies are called derogatory names in the hope that this will avert the evil eye, or they are given secret names which no-one else may pronounce and which they may not be told about until they are adult. Even though they may have a formal name, they may be called by a family or nickname which embodies certain

characteristics or might even refer to the particular circumstances of birth.

EXCLUSION AND PURIFICATION

In almost every culture, women who have just given birth
are excluded from normal work for at least a few days, with
more or less formal ritual. A Yukaghir woman in Siberia
must not touch anything in the house for three days. On the
fourth day, the midwife washes her and she in turn washes
the midwife's hands, wiping them with fresh shavings of
willow or a piece of newly prepared reindeer skin. She is
then purified with smoke, dry grass being lit and the woman
passing through the smoke while shaking her body. After
this she can return to her normal household duties but she
is considered unclean for a total of forty days. She must not,
therefore, have sexual intercourse, neither must she touch or
have anything to do with hunting or fishing implements.
Gypsy women are not allowed to touch kitchen utensils or
prepare food for the four to six weeks until the baby has a
gypsy baptism. Only then will the father be able to kiss his
newborn child. Once this period of impurity is over the
woman washes herself in the river and everything she has
used since giving birth is either burnt or thrown away.

Massage and abdominal binding are important treatments
which women in traditional societies have to help them overcome the rigours of giving birth and get their bodies back to
normal. The Chukchee mother's hips are bound tightly with
a cord for three days to bring the bones back to the right
position. Immediately after birth, the Malay mother is massaged and her abdomen bound to encourage the organs to
return to their normal places. This massage and binding is
carried out for a minimum of three days but might continue
for the whole forty days of the *pantang* or exclusion period.
A week or so after giving birth she may be massaged with a
special ball made of metal or stone. This is heated on the
fire and wrapped in a cloth and then rolled around on her
abdomen.

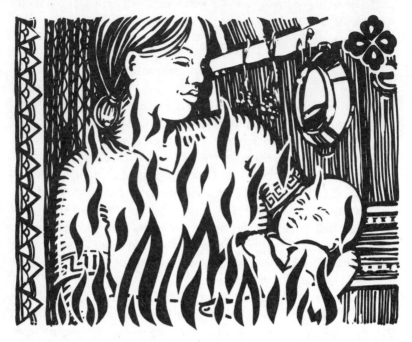

In south east Asia, the custom of sitting mothers by a fire for a period of time after giving birth, which is sometimes known as 'roasting', used to be very popular and is also found in many other parts of the word. In Thailand this fire is made with special smokeless wood which has been collected by the husband for this purpose during his wife's pregnancy. Sometimes, the woman just sits close to the fire while in some places there is a special bed made with the fire actually underneath it. As well as keeping the mother warm, the smoke is also thought to purify her and keep away evil spirits.

In the heat of the equatorial climate of south east Asia I used to wonder how any woman could bear to do this when it was already so hot. When I asked about this I was told that whether the woman does this or not depends on how she feels. Generally, it is carried out much less often and for shorter periods than it used to be but if she is very exhausted, at night and at certain times of the year, it can be very comforting. Most mothers, however, do keep themselves warm by wearing extra clothes and woollen socks and only drinking hot drinks. I caused considerable consternation after the birth of my daughter by walking around the house in bare feet and eating food and drink straight from the refrigerator. Older women friends in particular clicked their teeth and said I would be lucky if I did not suffer from pains in my joints when I got older!

Food is a very important item for the mother at this time and some cultures have very elaborate prescriptions about what should and should not be eaten. The Thai mother is considered to be very weak and exhausted, with her uterus full of harmful fluids. Heat is needed to warm her and give her the power to 'push out the fluids'. This is provided by the fire but also by the hot water that she both bathes in and drinks copiously. She eats only 'safe' basic foods like rice and takes 'hot' medicine to make her as hot as possible and therefore encourage the winds within her body to move and expel the fluids.

The Malay mother is thought to enter a very 'cold' phase after giving birth so that she too must watch her diet and eat only foods that will heat up her body to its normal level. In some places, the mother has to eat a very bland diet of only rice and salt water for a few days in order to expel all the blood. Special foods to increase lactation may be given and women may continue to eat these throughout the whole period of breastfeeding.

I asked what treatment was given to women who had suffered perineal tears during birth. Many people told me that women did not suffer from this problem and that this was something they had never seen. At first I thought they had not understood the question, but even after further explanation, many told me that this rarely happened. After my experience in the west where nearly everyone I knew either had an episiotomy or a tear, I found this difficult to believe. They did, however, have an explanation for this; either that the women were very active and healthy so that the tissue stretched easily, or that the babies were born slowly so that the perineum had time to stretch sufficiently without tearing.

One Malay midwife I spoke to did have a treatment which consisted of honey into which a special nut had been rubbed. She said she put some on the tear for as long as it took to heal and then gave the woman the rest to drink to heal the insides of her body. However, even she said that it was a very exceptional thing to happen and she rarely needed to use this treatment.

In parts of Africa, especially where female circumcision is undertaken, the birth attendant may have no choice but to cut the perineum if the baby is to be born. These cuts are often a source of infection and in some cases cause considerable further problems with the woman's urinary tract which only modern surgery is capable of curing.

BREASTFEEDING

In traditional societies all mothers breastfeed and there is an assumption that every mother can and will do so. In all the places I visited, I came across no-one who had been unable to breastfeed or who knew of anyone who had failed to provide enough breastmilk for their baby. For girls growing up in such a society, breastfeeding is an everyday activity which they see going on around them and so they learn the techniques unconsciously at an early age.

The period of rest and seclusion after birth provides a time of relative calm and support during which breastfeeding can be established. Many cultures, however, consider that colostrum, the fluid expressed by the breasts in the first two days after birth, is either irrelevant or bad for the baby. It may either be expressed by hand and discarded or the newborn just waits until the mother starts producing milk. During this time the baby may be given a substitute, sometimes sugar or honey mixed with water, although I was told by many of the women I spoke to that they gave the baby to another breastfeeding woman. Interestingly, several women told me that this was only necessary after the birth of the first baby when 'there was no milk in the breasts'. During the pregnancy of the second child, during which they would probably continue breastfeeding their first, there would be milk in the breasts and they assumed that this was available for the new baby as soon as he or she was born. I was surprised that this early disruption of breastfeeding didn't impair their ability to do so, but it didn't seem to make any difference. Perhaps the assumption that they would breastfeed was sufficient to overcome it.

There seemed to be very few problems experienced with breastfeeding and my questions as to how problems of lack of milk or cracked nipples would be dealt with were met with much discussion. There were remedies for lack of milk, but this was almost unheard of although they were often taken as a precautionary measure. The flower of a banana blossom was a remedy that I found throughout south east Asia, although the Batak in Sumatra said that raw peanuts were also very good. Chicken was thought to be a very strengthening thing to eat, both to overcome the rigours of childbirth and to increase lactation. I came across very few people for whom cracked nipples were a problem and only one group, the Karen, had a cure for it, consisting of the fat found under the shell of a land crab which had to be caught in the rice *padi*,

When the baby is first put to the breast, a small ceremony is often carried out either by the person who helped with the birth or a female relative. The Malays touch the baby's mouth with salt and then with gold and silver, but no-one I spoke to could remember the significance of this. The Karen give the baby a few grains of rice, symbolically telling her that this is what she will be eating in a year's time when she finishes breastfeeding.

WHEN THE BABY DIES

One of the most encouraging things about my research in south east Asia was the evidence I collected for the increasing number of healthy babies being born in many of the traditional villages that I visited. In most places, people thought they were healthier than they used to be and many mentioned how there were now fewer babies dying soon after birth. Better and more abundant food and clean water were the reasons generally given, together with the elimination of some unhealthy practices such as giving raw pork to children to eat; this was the cause of many fatal cases of worm infestation. As far as I could tell, the impact of western-type medical care on most of these people was negligible. In most cases they lived too far away from such medical facilities to benefit from them and usually it was far too expensive for them to afford.

This is not the case, of course, in some traditional societies where a combination of inadequate diet, poor water supply and an attitude towards women which means they are often malnourished leads to high neonatal death rates. In Bangladesh, for instance, which has one of the highest neonatal death rates in the world, the cycle that produces this starts at birth. A girl has less value than a boy and as a result has less food and later is less likely to be sent to school. She will be married early to reduce the number of dependents at home and although the legal age of marriage is eighteen, a girl is considered ready for marriage by the time she first menstruates and the average age for bearing the first baby is seventeen. An adult female is the last to eat in any household and her special nutritional needs during pregnancy and breast-feeding are not recognized. Cultural taboos discourage her from eating many nutritious foods, as it is generally believed that the smaller the baby, the easier the delivery. Given that many mothers are either young or have suffered a lifetime of malnutrition, this is probably a reasonable belief. Bangladeshi mothers given birth to babies of low birthweight which are more likely to die or to perpetuate the problems of illness, especially in the context of the poverty in which most of them live.

When a baby dies soon after birth it may be a reflection of the poverty and difficult circumstances in which the family finds itself, or it could be seen as the result of evil forces at work. Maybe the parents took insufficient care during pregnancy and birth, and sometimes, as amongst the Bu in Africa, the woman or man may be accused of killing the child. In this case a ceremony must be undertaken to exorcise their guilt, otherwise future pregnancies will be put in jeopardy. More often, however, the cause is seen as being outside the control of the parents, as spirits or evil magic were used to snatch the baby's soul away before it had a chance to live.

For a baby to be born, however, does not imply that it is fully human. Often, babies that die soon after birth are considered never to have lived and, in some cases, this is thought to show that they were some kind of spirit. This is often reflected in the lack of ceremony with which a dead baby is buried or otherwise disposed of.

Babies that do not conform to a particular idea of being human, in that they are deformed or multiple births, may not be allowed to live. Somewhat less commonly, babies are killed if the birth is illegitimate or if the mother dies in childbirth. In some places, there is also a certain amount of female infanticide, especially when food is short. Babies that exhibit various characteristics believed to show that they are witches or otherwise evil must also be killed. Sometimes, as amongst the Benin in Africa, it is the mother's responsibility to identify and kill such babies, but in others the whole groups is involved. If twins are born to a mother in an Akkha village in northern Thailand, they must be killed immediately and the whole village is involved in a series of complicated rituals to protect everyone from the evil of which the twins were a manifestation.

These practices have usually been roundly condemned as inhuman and horrible by members of our society. In the west, once a baby has been born and is breathing he or she is considered a full human being worth of protection from parents and the rest of society. To kill a baby in this situation is therefore considered murder. Amongst traditional societies, however, this is not necessarily the case as being deformed, being a twin or having some other characteristic indicative of evil also shows that it is not human and therefore not worthy of protection as such.

In most traditional societies, if the baby is to be killed it must either not be allowed to breathe or be killed very soon after birth. Once the baby has become a legitimate human

being, through having lived for a certain period after birth
or being named, then killing it becomes impossible. The
question seems to me to be one of definition, and the way
in which we define 'human' is rather different to the way in
which it is defined in other places. The widespread use of
pre-natal testing in western societies to identify and then
abort deformed babies seems to me very similar to the killing
of a deformed newborn baby. Why is the latter any more
repugnant than the former?

DEALING WITH PROBLEMS

Once the exclusion period is finished, mothers usually have
few problems. They do not suffer the isolation of the modern
woman or, usually, the full responsibility of bringing up their
baby. They will have help from female relatives and friends
so that the hard work of bringing up a baby can be shared.
In the close network of relationships and support that a
traditional society provides, there are rarely problems for the
new mother in adjusting to her role.

Sometimes, however, a woman may suffer with what in
the west we would call post-natal depression, although I
came across no cases of this. The baby cries incessantly, the
mother is irritable, loses her appetite, can't sleep and cries
for no reason. In Malaysia this is thought to be caused by a
hantu meroyan (a sort of ghost or spirit) interfering with the
normal course of the puerperium. Mothers who have been
saddened or angered during the post-partum period are said
to suffer from this more often.

For mild cases, a *bomoh* or traditional doctor is called to
treat the case with incantations and magically treated water
and prayers. If this doesn't work then a spirit-raising ceremony, or *main puteri* will be conducted with a shaman, his
assistant, a drummer and player of cymbals being engaged
for the three evenings on which the ritual takes place. The
shaman goes into a trance and first takes on the persona of
the inner forces or guardians of both his and his patient's
body. Through them he strengthens and restores her *semangat*

or spirit. Various *hantu* or spirits are then persuaded to speak through the shaman's mouth and to respond to his questioning to find out which of them is responsible for the woman's condition. When the offending *hantu* is found, it is cajoled or bribed into leaving. After this the woman is encouraged to go into a trance when she can express any emotion she likes; laughing, crying, singing, dancing and even flirting with the *bomoh* are all acceptable. When she emerges from this experience she is greeted with the approval of the family and friends who have been watching the ceremony. The opportunity to express unexpressed emotions in an appropriate and unthreatening atmosphere with concern for her being shown by everyone is usually sufficient to cure the problem.

INTRODUCTION OF THE NEWBORN TO THE WORLD

In many cultures there are special ceremonies which formally introduce the newborn to the society in which she is to live. In Russia, when a baby was christened according to the Russian Orthodox Church, this was done three days after birth. The family went to the river for 'holy water' which was sprinkled around the house and then drunk by the family on the morning of the christening. The doors, windowsills and front gate were marked with crosses; originally by children but in recent times more often by adults. After the ceremony, there was a christening feast with a special porridge being served by the midwife who received thanks in the form of small change from everyone. The infant would also be presented with gifts to 'teethe on'.

In Haiti the baby is introduced to the world by the midwife three days after the cord drops off. With water and candle in her hand she takes the child and presents her to the sun and then to the four corners of the earth with suitable incantations. She then takes her to the courtyard of the house; later there is also a ceremony when the baby is taken across the threshold for the first time. In Malaysia, after the forty day exclusion period, the midwife takes the baby down the steps of the house. She has with her a tray on which is iron, gold and silver. First she puts the feet of the child on each of these substances before putting the feet on the ground. All these ceremonies show that a mother has once again successfully given birth and that a new member of the group has arrived.

CHAPTER FIVE

BIRTH TODAY AND TOMORROW

•

What can we learn from these birth traditions? The ideas and approaches seem so different that it is very difficult to find points of contacts between traditional and western practices. The woman in the west expects to receive medical care during her pregnancy and the vast majority go to hospital to give birth. This would probably not matter if pregnancy and birth were viewed as normal processes but her experience of antenatal care will include being screened for problems and maybe being told that she is part of a 'high risk' group and therefore more likely to develop them. She will, either explicitly or implicitly, be expected to defer to the doctor's ideas as to what is good for her and the responsibility for finding and dealing with problems will be the doctor's rather than hers.

In traditional societies, pregnancy and birth are normal processes central to the life and identity of a woman. A pregnant woman receives advice and care from female relatives and friends and has access to the help of a more experienced traditional midwife or other traditional specialist should she need it. She protects herself not only physically but, with various rituals, spiritually as well, some of the rituals marking various stages of the pregnancy as the time for giving birth approaches. She harnesses positive forces to protect both her and the unborn baby; focuses on various images through what she eats and what she does that will clear the way in her body so that the baby can be born easily. The responsibility for the baby will be hers alone although she will be supported by her husband and, more importantly, other women who will affirm her unique position as the bearer of a new life.

When the time comes to give birth the women from a traditional society may do so completely on her own or with the help and support of other women. Her husband may or may not be present at birth, but he will participate in the birth in the ways approved by that culture, although his role will be secondary unless there are problems which he may have to help resolve. Birth takes place in quiet and seclusion, either at home or in a special place set aside for the purpose. The moment of birth is a time of great significance.

By contrast, the women in the west will go to hospital to give birth and will suffer all the problems of doing so in an impersonal institution; she will have little privacy, will not know her birth attendants and will in all probability be moved around at different stages of labour. Many hospitals are, of course, trying to change this environment and a few have successfully managed to do so. I do not minimize the difficulties of trying to provide a personal and sensitive service in a large institution which is basically impersonal and insensitive. All too often, however, the changes made are only cosmetic and the basic institutional approach and attitudes of the staff remain the same. The woman giving birth will have to defer to the medical personnel's idea of what is good for her and may come under intense pressure to receive analgesics and to submit to other interventions 'for the good of herself and her baby'. The medical personnel's main consideration will be the safe extraction of a healthy baby and to this end the mother's feelings about what is happening to her are likely to be ignored and in many cases completely dismissed.

Once the baby has been born the woman in hospital will be moved yet again to another ward where she may stay for a few hours or days before going home. Although there are community midwives and health visitors who may visit her for a time she will, in all probability, be very much on her own in caring for the baby. If she has younger children or if she needs to work, she may feel very strongly that she must get up and be 'back to normal' as soon as possible, however she feels. Compared to women in a traditional society, for a woman in the west this time after birth is very rushed and gives her little time and opportunity to adjust to the immense changes which have taken place within her, and to her new responsibilities as a mother.

Immediately after birth, in a traditional society, there is a time of rest and seclusion for the new mother and this period is also often a time when she is not allowed to carry out any domestic duties. There will be various rituals connected with the placenta and the protection of the newborn and she may have to eat special food to regain her strength and increase her milk supply for the baby. She can be assured of help and support from her female relatives and friends and later, when she does resume her normal household work, it will be in their company and with their help in looking after the newborn.

This may perhaps seem a rather idealized account given that many women in third world countries are very poor and must work hard to support their families; if they cannot work then the family may starve. This time of seclusion after birth, however, is considered extremely important and takes precedence over all other considerations. As I found during my research, even in the most deprived circumstances families rally round to ensure that women who have just given birth have this time of recuperation, even though it may have to be shortened or the rituals involved kept to a minimum.

In recent years, one of the most important things that we have rediscovered from traditional ideas is giving birth in an upright position. Until the mid-seventeenth century women had always given birth either standing, squatting or kneeling and anything used to help them do this, such as a rope hanging from the ceiling or a birthing chair, did not disturb or change this.

The first woman to give birth lying on her back was a mistress of the French King Louis IX who assumed this position so that her lover could watch the birth from behind a screen. The invention of the forceps by the Chamberlain brothers in France during the seventeenth century encouraged more women to lie on their backs to give birth as forceps, which were at first shrouded in secrecy, could only be used if the woman was lying on her back. It became the fashion for ladies of quality to give birth lying on their backs while at the same time the male obstetrician took over the conduct of the birth from the female midwife.

Giving birth with the use of anaesthetics, such as the chloroform first used by Queen Victoria, further intensified the use of the recumbent position. Every technological advance since then, in particular induction and various forms of foetal monitoring, have intensified this process and with it the passivity and controllability of the women giving birth. As birth became less of a natural function supported by women and more of a medical problem controlled by men, women were encouraged to ignore their deepest instincts about giving birth and lie down for the convenience of their birth attendants.

The vast majority of women in traditional societies give birth in an upright position and there are very good reasons for doing so. In this position the pelvic opening through which the baby is born is at its widest and shortest, especially if the woman squats. The heavy weight of the baby and the placenta are not lying on the large blood vessels that run by the spine, which is what happens when the mother gives birth lying down. Being upright greatly increases the blood flow to the baby through the placenta thus increasing the baby's oxygen supply during the crucial period of birth.

Standing, sitting or squatting uses the forces of gravity more effectively; the pressure of the baby's head on the cervix is greater, thus increasing the strength and effectiveness of the uterine contractions. Mechanically, it is much more advantageous to push the baby out towards the earth than to push it along the horizontal as must be done when the woman lies on her back. As the baby is born, the pressure on the perineum is spread more evenly and it is thus much less likely to tear and if it does so, the tear is unlikely to be very deep or serious. The benefits in terms of how the woman feels are also considerable as she is usually much more comfortable and the pain is less. I felt a great sense of power and independence in giving birth with two feet firmly on the ground and I don't think this feeling is unusual in women who give birth in this way.

I think it is interesting that, in the wake of this increasing use of a 'new' upright position in which to give birth, has come a proliferation of birthing chairs and tables. These are often advertised as enabling the women who use them to assume the 'right' position in which to give birth, as well as being designed for the convenience of birth attendants. I suppose such devices are better than the old form of delivery tables but it seems to me as yet another form of control. A woman must still be 'engineered' into the right position for birth rather than being left to find the right position for herself when the time comes.

Each woman is different and will use whatever positions she needs for her own comfort and convenience; there is an infinite variety and she must have the freedom to choose what is right for her rather than be forced into a prescribed pattern or position. This requires a shift in the attitudes of the birth attendants rather than a change in the nature of the equipment. I cannot help feeling that, yet again, it is the demands of the medical establishment and the market which are being met rather than the real needs of labouring women. There are, of course, far more profits to be made from selling birthing chairs of a complicated design than lengths of rope or even cushions which are far cheaper and infinitely more adjustable to the needs of individuals.

Often, the people who ask me what the west can learn from traditional societies are thinking in terms of techniques or remedies that we might use. Everywhere I went there were local remedies to deal with the common problems of pregnancy and the fact that they were local was, of course, their main advantage. The coconut water that the Indonesian mother uses, often in conjunction with suitable religious rituals, to help her morning sickness is freely available from the many coconut trees that grow around most Indonesian villages. Similarly, the bamboo that the Malay midwife used to cut the umbilical cord grows everywhere and it is simplicity itself to cut a sliver when the time comes and then to dispose of it after the birth.

It is ironic that we should now be asking about these methods when in the past and even nowadays, biomedical methods are being imposed on traditional societies often by governments anxious to implement a modern western type of medical system. I have come across several instances in the literature of indigenous practices which were condemned just because they did not conform to the biomedical view-point. These include such things as the kind of instruments which should be used to cut the umbilical cord as well as what constitutes a 'good diet'. Before biomedical doctors condemn such practices they would do well to look at their own record of techniques which have been offered to preg-nant women. The history of pregnancy care in the last fifty years or so is littered with the use of drugs and procedures which, although seen at the time as helpful, have sub-sequently been found to be, at best, useless or, at worst, downright dangerous. Traditional techniques and remedies have evolved and been tested over many thousands of years and while some are certainly harmful, they cannot all be condemned. Often they are efficacious and usually they have the added advantage of being cheap and accessible to anyone who wants to use them.

To answer the question in this way, however, and to look for no more than remedies or techniques which can be added to our repertoire of cures in the west is, I believe, to miss the real lessons which we need to learn. Asking and answer-ing the question in this way is to implicitly assume a biomed-ical perspective. It is all too easy to assume that biomedicine is a superior and advanced form of medicine to which a few traditional remedies and techniques can be grafted. As I hope this book has shown, biomedicine is based on a certain idea about the body and the mind and its connections. It leads us to view the mind as separate from the body which works rather like a machine, but there is nothing inherently superior about this view or the kind of medicine which derives from it. This is not to belittle the benefits which biomedicine can bestow, especially in the treatment of infections, diseases and some conditions requiring surgery. In the case of the care which is provided for pregnancy and birth, however, this is physically based and not necessarily always appropriate.

Of course, part of the reason why these medical ideas have had such an impact on pregnancy care in the west is that pregnancy and birth have come to be seen as a medical problem requiring a medical solution. In traditional societies, pregnancy and birth are viewed as normal conditions which, although there may be certain vulnerabilities and dangers, are not especially hazardous. By comparison, the biomedical view is that pregnancy and birth are potentially very danger-ous conditions which can only be dealt with by professionally qualified medical personnel. As Sally Inch commented, 'Pro-fessionals who believe that every birth is a potential death which can only be averted by their ministrations will nat-urally be reluctant to relinquish any area of control over the process.' In the last fifty years pregnancy and birth have come to be viewed as pathology rather than a naturally occurring process.

While biomedicine does have a predominantly physical focus, in recent years there has been an upsurge of interest and research trying to determine how body and mind interact and the implications this has for our health. Generally, this has focused on the immune system and the balance of hor-mones, blood, brain and nervous activity which enables us to repel infection and remain healthy. At the same time, it has also given us insights as to how the healthy balance of the body is maintained through the control that the hypo-thalamus exerts on unconscious bodily processes such as heartbeat, blood pressure and digestion. Known as the 'primal system' of our bodies, it is this which controls the process of giving birth and which, it has been found, both affects and is affected by our mental processes, in particular by images. Imagery has been used for many years in psycho-therapy and is now being used to an increasing degree to promote health. Most of the work being done is with people who are ill with either incurable or chronic diseases and there is, of course, resistance on the part of some biomedical doctors to accept and use these ideas.

As we have seen, in traditional societies imagery is used in many ways by pregnant women to both protect themselves and prepare themselves for giving birth. What a woman does, what she eats and the rituals that she undertakes are all opportunities for symbolically influencing both herself and her unborn baby. In the west we have forgotten the language of images, preferring instead to concentrate on analytical and explanatory modes of thought and communication. These are very necessary, of course, but are inadequate for communicating with ourselves and for viewing ourselves and our situations in a holistic way. I think we should learn from women in traditional societies and find ways of using images to get in touch with and trust that primal part of ourselves, the working of which is so necessary to give birth efficiently. Images can be used to change bodily processes and we too should use these to help us give birth. Clearing doorways and untying knots are images used by pregnant women the world over, but we must also find our own which may well derive from our experience of life in western society.

While I was pregnant with my third child I used the Malaysian idea of open doors and windows – whenever I saw one I thought of my baby coming out easily. As it happens she did! I think that the images one uses have to be meaningful to the person who uses them so that everyone has to find their own and what works best for them. I would love to hear from pregnant women as to what images they have used – either consciously or unconsciously – to find which ones are most prevalent and meaningful in our society.

Individual preparations of this nature, however, cannot on their own bring about the radical shift of consciousness which I think is necessary to change the way in which we give birth in the west. While we continue to give birth in hospitals where the ethos and physical focus are so different and where power rests with the medical establishment rather than the woman giving birth, then real change is impossible. In her book on the history of antenatal care Ann Oakley says that we have now come to a crucial point where we have to choose between two sorts of care for pregnant and labouring women. We can continue with an even greater accelerated technical growth and accompanying depersonalization and dehumanization which have marked these services since such technology was introduced. Or we can reinstate antenatal care as a social concern, sensitive to the psychosocial needs of families and recognizing the wisdom of women and parents.

Of course, many hospitals have tried to make themselves more 'patient sensitive' but pot plants in the waiting room and curtains in the delivery room do not a patient-sensitive system make. So often, these are only cosmetic changes and the underlying attitudes remain the same. I cannot see how this will ever change unless we demedicalize pregnancy and birth completely and give the responsibility for birth back to women, where it has always been until recently. There will always be some women, of course, who require medical care but the proportion is very small. Opinions vary on this proportion, but any figure given must take into account those women who need assistance because of problems caused by medical intervention at an earlier stage of pregnancy or birth. What justification can there be for keeping antenatal care as part of medical services when such a small proportion of women need medical care and when, for normal women, it does more harm than good? Why should women have to submit to medical care when they don't need it, especially when this in itself destroys the confidence and support which normal women need to give birth successfully?

Taking pregnancy services out of the medical context is the only way of overcoming these problems as well as recognizing birth as the social and spiritual event that it is. At the same time, pregnancy and birth care should be provided by women; that is, by midwives rather than obstetricians. Birth could take place either at home or in local birth centres and only those suffering from recognized medical complications would go to hospital. This would only be a small number of women, who would be able to take the local midwife with them as well as family and friends for support.

The birth centre could be a focus for anyone bringing

up children, serving the same supportive function which is provided informally by women in traditional societies. A place to eat, to share experiences and to provide mutual support and help which is as important as professional help and advice. There would be far more 'direct entry' midwives who had not been nurses first, including older women who, having enjoyed the births of their own children, would want to share their experiences. Fewer obstetricians would be needed, but they would have to be not only competent doctors but also very special people. Those who would participate in the mystery of birth must be especially sensitive, particularly when they are dealing with women who are not only giving birth but also experiencing problems in doing so.

The way in which we have come to care for pregnant and labouring women in the west is, I believe, a reflection of the general way in which we live which has brought us to this present environmental crisis. We live as if the world is ours to use as we like and that we can take from it with no thought of the balance we are disturbing or the damage we are creating. We assume that we can control the world with what we think of as our superior intellect, just as we assume that the process of birth can be managed and controlled by external means or by an act of conscious will.

The irony is that the more we try to control natural processes and ignore natural systems and balances, the more we destroy and the less real control we are able to exercise. This is certainly true for women giving birth in the west who take less responsibility for themselves and have far less control over what happens to them than a woman giving birth in a traditional society. Because of all the paraphernalia of modern obstetrical care, she is often completely alienated from the deep primitive instincts from which the real power to give birth is derived. Our older birth traditions affirm and support these powerful forces and stem from a different and more humble view of the place that we as humans have in the world. In this context birth is not just a physical process to be controlled but a complex mystery of forces which must be allowed to progress in their natural way. Only in exceptional circumstances will problems occur and only then will intervention be right and necessary.

It is this view of birth which really distinguishes traditional from western practices and that an understanding of our birth traditions can help us appreciate. Changing our view of birth is not only a necessary precursor for making necessary changes in the care we give to pregnant and labouring women. It is part of the shift in consciousness which must take place if the human cycle of birth and death is to continue into the twenty-first century.

REFERENCES

•

CHAPTER 1

1. Granquist, H. *Birth and Childhood among the Arabs: Studies in a Muhammadan Village in Palestine.* Sodestrom & Co., 1947.
2. Muecke, M. 'Health care systems as socialising agents: child-bearing the North Thai and western ways.' *Social Science and Medicine,* Vol. 10; pp. 377–83.

CHAPTER 2

1. Laderman, C. *Wives and Midwives: Childbirth and Nutrition in Rural Malaysia.* University of California Press, 1983.
2. Maurer, D. & Maurer, C. *The World of the Newborn.* Penguin, 1988.
3. Granquist, H. See above.
4. Longo, L. D. 'Sociocultural practices relating to obstetrics and gynecology in a community of West Africa.' *Obstetrics and Gynecology in West Africa,* Vol. 39, 4; pp. 470–5.
5. Rowland, B. *The Medieval Woman's Guide to Health: The First English Gynecological Handbook.* (p 32) Kent State University Press, 1981.
6. Hall, M. H. 'An Appraisal of Outpatient Antenatal Care in Aberdeen', unpublished paper described in Oakley, A. *The Captured Womb.* Basil Blackwell, 1984.

CHAPTER 3

1. Tupper, C. 'Conditioning for childbirth.' *American Journal of Obstetrics and Gynecology*, April 1956; pp 733–40.
2. Van Auken, W. B. D., Tomlinson, D. R. & Troy, N. Y. 'An appraisal of patient training for childbirth.' *American Journal of Obstetrics and Gynecology*, Vol. 66, 1.
3. Copstick, S., Kayes, R. W., Taylor, K. E. & Morris, N. 'A test of common assumptions regarding the use of antenatal training during labour.' *Journal of Psychosomatic Research*, Vol. 29, 2; pp 215–18.
4. Odent, M. *Primal Health*. Century Hutchinson, 1986.
5. Brown, A. 'Fathers in Labour Wards: Medical and Lay Accounts', in McKee, L. & O'Brien, M. (eds) *The Father Figure*, Tavistock, 1982.
6. Garforth, S. & Garcia, J. 'Admitting – a weakness or a strength? Routine admission of women in labour.' *Midwifery*, Vol. 3; pp 10–24.
7. Campbell, A. 'Birth Indian style.' *Midwives' Chronicle and Nursing Notes*, Vol. 103, 1; p 227.
8. Moore, R. 'Ethnographic assessment of pain coping perceptions.' *Psychosomatic Medicine*, Vol. 52; pp 156–70.
9. Waldenstrom, U. 'Midwives' attitudes to pain relief during labour and delivery.' *Midwifery*, Vol. 4; pp 48–57.
10. Siegal, B. *Peace, Love and Healing*. Century Hutchinson, 1990.
11. Achterberg, J. *Imagery and Healing: Shamanism and Modern Medicine*. New Science Library, Shambhala, 1985.
12. Tew, M. 'The practices of birth attendants and the safety of birth.' *Midwifery*, Vol. 2; pp 3–10.
13. Damstra-Wijmenga, S. M. I. 'Home confinement: the positive results in Holland.' *Journal of the Royal College of General Practitioners*, August 1984; pp 425–31.
14. Cronk, M. & Flint, C. *Community Midwifery – A Practical Guide*. Heinemann Nursing, 1989.

CHAPTER 4

1. Gerdel, F. 'A case of delayed afterbirth among the Tzeltal Indians.' *American Anthropologist*, Vol. 51; p 158.
2. Gordon, J. E., Gideon, H. & Wyon, J. B. 'Midwifery practices

in the Punjab, India.' *American Journal of Obstetrics and Gynecology*, **Vol.** 93, 5; pp 735–43.

3. Botha, M. G. 'The management of the umbilical cord in labour.' *South African Journal of Obstetrics and Gynaecology*, **Vol.** 6, 2; pp 662–7. Described in Inch, S. 'Management of the third stage of labour – another cascade of intervention?' *Midwifery*, **Vol.** 1; pp 114–22.

4. Begley, C. M. 'A comparison of "active" and "physiological" management of third stage of labour.' *Midwifery*, **Vol.** 6; pp 3–17.

BIBLIOGRAPHY

•

Achterberg, J. *Imagery and Healing; Shaminism and Modern Medicine*. New Science Library, Shambhala, 1985.

Ader, R. 'Developmental psychoneuroimmunology.' *Developmental Psychobiology*, Vol. 16, 4; pp 251–67.

Antle, May, K. 'The three phases of father involvement in pregnancy.' *Nursing Research*, Vol. 31, 6; pp 337–42.

Antle May, K. & Perrin, S. P. 'Prelude: Pregnancy and Birth', from Hanson, S. M. H. & Bozett, F. W. (eds) *Dimensions of Fatherhood*. Saga Publications, 1985.

Asuni, T. 'Modern Medicine and Traditional Medicine', from Ademuwagun, Z. A., Ayoade, J. A. A. Harrison, I. E. & Warren, D. M. (eds) *African Therapeutic Systems*. Crossroads Press, 1979.

Awang Hasmadi Awang Mois. 'Beliefs and practices concerning births among the Selako of Sarawak.' *Sarawak Museum Journal*, Vol. XXVI, 47; pp 7–13.

Balaskas, J. *New Active Birth*. Thorsons 1991.

Baudesson, H. *Indochina and Its Primitive Peoples*. Hutchinson and Co.

Beardsley, R. K., Hall, J. W. & Ward, R. E. *Village Japan*. University of Chicago Press, 1959.

Beck, N. C. *et al.* 'Preparation for labour: a historical perspective'. *Psychosomatic Medicine*, Vol. 41, 3; pp 243–58.

Beck, N. C. & Siegel, L. J. 'Preparation for childbirth and contemporary research on pain, anxiety, and stress reduction: a review and critique.' *Psychosomatic Medicine*, Vol. 42, 4; pp 429–47.

Beck, N. C. & Hall, D. 'Natural childbirth: a review and analysis.' *Obstetrics and Gynecology*, Vol. 52, 3; pp 371–9.

Begley, C. M. 'A comparison of "active" and "physiological" management of third stage of labour.' *Midwifery*, Vol. 6; pp 3–17.

138   BIRTH TRADITIONS

Bell, D. *Daughters of the Dreaming*. George Allen and Unwin, 1983.
Blackman, W. S. *The Fellahin of Upper Egypt*. Frank Cass and Co., 1968.
Blake, R. *Mind over Medicine*. Pan Books, 1987.
Blalock, E. 'The immune system as a sensory organ.' *Journal of Immunology*, 1984; pp 1067–70.
Borysenko, J. *Minding the Body, Mending the Mind*. Bantam Books, 1988.
Breslow, L. 'A quantitative approach to World Health Organization definition of health; physical, mental and social wellbeing.' *International Journal of Epidemiology*, Vol. 1, 4; pp 347–55.
Brown, A. 'Fathers in the labour ward: medical and lay accounts', from McKee, L. & O'Brien, M. (eds) *The Father Figure*. Tavistock, 1982.
Campbell, A. 'Birth Indian Style.' *Midwives Chronicle and Nursing Notes*, Vol. 103, 1; p 227.
Cannon, W. B. 'Voodoo death.' *Psychosomatic Medicine*, Vol. 14, 3; pp 183–90.
Chapekar, L. N. *Thakurs of the Sahyadri*. Oxford University Press, 1960.
Clebert, J. P. *The Gypsies*. (English translation) Vista Books, 1963.
Cogan, R. 'Comfort during prepared childbirth as a function of parity, reported by four classes of participant observers.' *Journal of Psychosomatic Research*, Vol. 19; pp 33–7.
Cominsky, S. 'Cross-cultural perspectives in Midwifery', from Grollig, Francis and Haley (eds) *Medical Anthropology*. Mouton Publishers, The Hague, 1976.
Copstick, S., Hawes, R. W., Taylor, K. E. & Morris, N. F. 'A test of common assumptions regarding the use of antenatal training during labour.' *Journal of Psychosomatic Research*, Vol. 29, 2; pp 215–18.
Cornell, J. B. & Smith, R. J. *Two Japanese Villages*. University of Michigan Press, 1956.
Cronenwett, L. R. & Newmark, L. L. 'Fathers' responses to childbirth.' *Nursing Research*, Vol. 23, 3; pp 210–16.
Cronk, M. & Flint, C. *Community Midwifery – A Practical Guide*. Heinemann Nursing, 1989.
Czaplicka, M. A. *Aboriginal Siberia: A Study in Social Anthropology*. Clarendon Press, 1969.
Damstra-Wijmenga, S. M. I. 'Home confinement: the positive

results in Holland.' *Journal of the Royal College of General Practitioners*, August 1984, pp 425–31.

Davids, A. & DeVault, S. 'Maternal anxiety during pregnancy and childbirth abnormalities.' *Psychosomatic Medicine*, Vol. 34, 5; pp 465–70.

Deng, F. M. *The Dinka of the Sudan*. Holt, Rinehart and Winston, 1972.

Dunn, S. P. & Dunn, E. *The Peasants of Central Russia*. Holt, Rinehart and Winston, 1967.

Ehrenreich, B. & English, D. *For Her Own Good: 150 Years of the Experts Advice to Women*. Pluto Press, 1988.

Ehrenreich, B. & English, D. *Witches, Midwives and Nurses: A History of Women Healers*. The Feminist Press, 1973.

Engel, G. 'The need for a new medical model: a challenge for biomedicine.' *Science*, Vol. 196, 4286, pp 129–36.

Evans-Pritchard, E. E. *Man and Woman Among the Azande*. Faber and Faber, 1974.

Field, M. J. *Religion and Medicine of the Ga People*. Oxford University Press, 1937.

Firth, R. *Tikopia Ritual and Belief*. George Allen and Unwin, 1967.

Fischer, A. 'Reproduction in Truk.' *Ethnology*, Vol. 2, pp 526–40.

Ford, C. S. 'A comparative study of human reproduction.' *Yale University Publications in Anthropology*, Vol. 32, pp 1–111.

Freedman, E. A. & Sachleben, M. R. 'Dysfunctional labour.' *Obstetrics and Gynecology*, Vol. 17, 2; pp 135–49.

Garforth, S. & Garcia, J. 'Admitting – a weakness or a strength? Routine admission of women in labour.' *Midwifery*, Vol. 3; pp 10–24.

Geertz, C. *The Religion of Java*. University of Chicago Press, 1960.

Gerdel, F. 'A case of delayed afterbirth among the Tzeltal Indians.' *American Anthropologist*, Vol. 51; 158.

Gibson, W. *Women in Seventeenth Century France*. Macmillan, 1989.

Gideon, H. 'A baby is born in the Punjab.' *American Anthropologist*', Vol. 64; pp 1220–34.

Glouberman, D. *Life Choices and Life Changes Through Imagework*. Mandala, Unwin Paperbacks, 1989.

Gordon, J. E. Gideon, H. & Wyon, J. B. 'Childbirth in rural Punjab, India.' *American Journal of Medical Sciences*, March 1964; pp 345–62.

Gordon, J. E., Gideon, H. & Wyon, J. B. 'Midwifery practices in the Punjab, India.' *American Journal of Obstetrics and Gynecology*, Vol. 93, 5; pp 735–43.

Granquist, H. *Birth and Childhood Among the Arabs: Studies in a Muhammadan Village in Palestine*. Sodestrom and Co., 1947.

Greenberg, M. & Morris, N. 'Engrossment: the newborn's impact upon the father.' *American Journal of Orthopsychiatry*, Vol. 44, 4; pp 520–31.

Gunter, L. M. 'Psychopathology and stress in the life experiences of mothers of premature infants.' *American Journal of Obstetrics and Gynecology*, June 1 1963; pp 333–40.

Harner, M. *The Way of the Shaman*. Bantam Books, 1982.

Henneborn, W. J. & Cogan, R. 'The effect of husband participation on reported pain and probability of medication during labour and birth.' *Journal of Psychosomatic Research*, Vol. 19; pp 215–22.

Hewat, M. L. *Bantu Folklore: Medical and General* (1906). Reprinted by Negro University Press 1970.

Huttel, F. A. *et al.* 'A quantitative evaluation of psychoprophylaxis in childbirth.' *Journal of Psychosomatic Research*, Vol. 16; pp 81–92.

Inch, S. 'Management of the third stage of labour – another cascade of intervention?' *Midwifery*, Vol. 1; pp 114–22.

Irvine, J. 'Changing patterns of social control in Buu society.' from Arens, W. (ed) *A Century of Change in Eastern Africa*. Mouton Publishers, 1976.

Jalland, P. & Hooper, J. *Women from Birth to Death: The Female Life Cycle in Britain 1830–1914*. The Harvester Press, 1986.

Jansen, W. *Women without Men: Gender and Marginality in an Algerian Town*. E. S. Brill, 1987.

Kendall, L. *Shamans, Housewives and Other Restless Spirits: Women in Korean Ritual*. University of Hawaii Press, 1985.

Kitzinger, S. *The Midwife Challenge*. Pandora Press, 1988.

Kleinman, A., Eisenberg, L. & Good, B. 'Culture, illness and care.' *Annals of Internal Medicine*, Vol. 88; pp 251–8.

Koss, J. D. 'The therapist-spiritist training project in Puerto Rico: an experiment to relate the traditional healing system to the public health system.' *Social Science and Medicine*, Vol. 14; pp 255–66.

Koss, J. D. 'Social process, healing and self-defeat among Puerto Rican spiritists.' *American Ethnologist* Vol. 4; pp 453–69.

Laderman, C. *Wives and Midwives: Childbirth and Nutrition in Rural Malaysia*. University of California Press, 1983.

Leather, E. M. *Folklore of Herefordshire.* undated.

Lederman, R. P. *et al.* 'The relationship of maternal anxiety, plasma catecholamines and plasma cortisol to progress in labour.' *American Journal of Obstetrics and Gynecology,* November 1st, 1978; pp 495–501.

Levi Strauss, C. *Structural Anthropology.* Basic Books, 1963.

Levy, R. I. 'Tahitian folk psychotherapy.' *International Mental Health Research Newsletter,* Vol. 9, 4; pp 12–15.

Lock, M. *East Asian Medicine in Urban Japan.* University of California Press, 1980.

Longo, L. D. 'Sociocultural practices relating to obstetrics and gynecology in a community of West Africa.' *Obstetrics and Gynecology in West Africa,* Vol. 89, 4; pp 470–75.

McClain, C. 'Ethno-Obstetrics in Ajijic.' *Anthropology Quarterly,* Vol. 48; pp 38–56.

Madan, T. N. *Family and Kinship: A Study of the Pandits of Rural Kashmir.* Asia Publishing House, 1965.

Maglaos, E. R. *The Potential of the Traditional Birth Attendant.* World Health Organization, 1986.

Maurer, D. & Maurer, C. *The World of the Newborn.* Penguin, 1988.

Meltzer, D. *Birth: An Anthology of Ancient Texts, Songs Prayers and Stories.* Northpoint Press, 1981.

Mendelson, M. Hirsch, S. & Webber, C. S. 'A critical examination of some recent theoretical models in psychosomatic medicine.' *Psychosomatic Medicine,* Vol. 18, 5; pp 363–73.

Mongeau, B., Smith, H. L. & Maney, A. 'The granny midwife: changing roles and functions of a folk practitioner.' *The American Journal of Sociology,* Vol. LXVI; pp 497–505.

Moors, R. 'Ethnographic assessment of pain coping mechanisms.' *Psychosomatic Medicine,* Vol. 52; pp 171–81.

Morris, N. 'Labour', from Donnerstein & Burrows (eds) *The Handbook of Psychosomatic Obstetrics and Gynaecology.* Elsevier Biomedical Press, 1983.

Muecke, M. 'Health care systems as socializing agents: childbearing the North Thai and western ways' *Social Science and Medicine,* Vol. 10; pp 377–83.

Mulcahy, R. A. & Janz, N. 'Effectiveness of raising pain perception thresholds in males and females using a psychoprophylactic childbirth technique during induced pain.' *Nursing Research,* Vol. 22, 5; pp 423–7.

Newton, N., Foshee, D. & Newton, M. 'Experimental inhibition of labour through environmental disturbance.' *Obstetrics and Gynecology*, Vol. 27, 3; pp 371–77.

Nicholson, S. *Shamanism: An Expanded View of Reality*. Quest Books, Theosophical Publishing House, 1987.

Oakley, A. *The Captured Womb: A History of the Medical Care of Pregnant Women*. Basil Blackwell, 1984.

Odent, M. *Primal Health*. Century Hutchinson, 1986.

Olbrechts, F. M. 'Cherokee belief and practice with regard to childbirth.' *Anthropos*, Vol. 26; pp 17–33.

Omer, H., Friedlander, D. & Palti, Z. 'Hypnotic relaxation in the treatment of premature labour.' *Psychosomatic Medicine*, Vol. 48, 5; pp 351–61.

Ortiz de Montellano, B. 'Empirical Aztec medicine.' *Science*, Vol. 188, 4185; pp 215–21.

Palmer, G. *The Politics of Breastfeeding*. Pandora Press, 1988.

Paul, L. 'The Mastery of Work and the Mystery of Sex in a Guatemalan Village', from Rosalde, M. Z. & Lamphere, L. (eds) *Women, Culture and Society*. Stanford University Press, 1974.

Paul, L. & Paul, B. 'The Maya midwife as sacred specialist: a Guatemalan case.' *American Ethnologist*, Vol. 2; pp 707–25.

Poole, F. J. P. 'Transforming "Natural" Woman: Female Ritual Leaders and Gender Ideology Among Bimin-Kuskusmin', from (eds) Ortner, S. B. & Whitehead, H. *Sexual Meanings: the Cultural Construction of Gender and Sexuality*. Cambridge University Press, 1981.

Porter, E. *Cambridgeshire Customs and Folklore*. Routledge and Kegan Paul, 1969.

Puckett, N. N. *Folk Beliefs of the Southern Negro*. Negro University Press, 1929.

Radford, E. & H. *Encyclopaedia of Superstitions*. Hutchinson and Sons, 1961.

Rajadhon, P. A. *Life and Ritual in Old Siam*. Hraf Press, 1961.

Randolf, V. *Ozark Magic and Folklore*. Dover Publications, 1947.

Rees, L. 'The development of psychosomatic medicine during the past 25 years.' *Journal of Psychosomatic Research*. Vol. 27, 2; pp 157–64.

Richardson Hanks, J. *Maternity and its Rituals in Bang Chan*. Cornell Thailand Project, Interim Report Series. No. 6; Data Paper No. 51. Southeast Asia Program, Cornell University, 1963.

Rivers, W. H. R. *The Todas*. Macmillan, 1906.

Roberts, H. *The Patient Patients: Women and their Doctors*. Pandora Press, 1985.

Rowland, B. *The Medieval Woman's Guide to Health: The First English Gynecological Handbook*. Kent State University Press, 1981.

Sargent, C. F. *Maternity, Medicine and Power: Reproductive Decisions in Urban Benin*. University of California Press, 1989.

Siegal, B. *Peace, Love and Healing*. Century Hutchinson, 1990.

Spencer, B. & Gillen, F. J. *The Native Tribes of Central Australia*. Macmillan and Co. 1899.

Spencer, R. F. 'Obstetrics and Population Control', from Landy, D. *Culture, Disease and Healing*. Macmillan Publishing, 1977.

Stacey, M. *The Sociology of Health and Healing*. Unwin Hyman, 1988.

Stevens, R. J. & Heide, F. 'Analgesic characteristics of prepared childbirth techniques: attention focusing and systematic relaxation.' *Journal of Psychosomatic Research*, **Vol. 21**; pp 429–38.

Suilleabmain, S. *Irish Folk Custom and Belief*. Three Candles, 1967.

Sutherland, A. *The Gypsies* Macmillan Publishing, 1975.

Tew, M. *Safer Childbirth? A Critical History of Maternity Care*. Chapman and Hall, 1990.

Tew, M. 'The practices of birth attendants and the safety of birth.' *Midwifery*, **Vol. 2**; pp 3–10.

Thompson, B. & Baird, Sir D. 'Some impressions of childbearing in tropical areas.' *Journal of Obstetrics and Gynaecology, British Commonwealth*, **Vol. 74**; pp 510–22.

Tupper, C. 'Conditioning for childbirth.' *American Journal of Obstetrics and Gynecology*, April 1956; pp 733–41.

Van Auken, W. B. D. & Tomlinson, D. R. 'An appraisal of patient training for childbirth.' *American Journal of Obstetrics and Gynecology*, **Vol. 66**, 1; pp 100–105.

Verny, T. and Kelly, J. *The Secret Life of the Unborn Child*. Sphere Books, 1982.

Villoldo, A. & Krippner, S. *Healing States*. Simon and Schuster, 1987.

Vincent Priya, J. *Birth Without Doctors* Earthscan, 1991.

Waldenstrom, U. 'Midwives' attitudes to pain relief during labour and delivery.' *Midwifery*, **Vol. 4**; pp 48–57.

Waring, P. *A Dictionary of Omens and Superstitions*. Souvenir Press, 1978.

Weiner, A. B. *The Trobrianders of Papua New Guinea*. Holt, Rinehard and Winston, 1988.

White, N. I. *The Frank C Brown Collection of North Carolina Folklore in Seven Volumes*. Duke University Press, 1961.

Wirz, P. *Exorcism and the Art of Healing in Ceylon*. E. S. Brill, 1954.

Wolf, M. *Women and the Family in Rural Taiwan*. Stanford University Press, 1972.

Worthington, E. L. 'Labour room and laboratory: clinical validation of the cold pressor as a means of testing preparation for childbirth strategies.' *Journal of Psychosomatic Research*, Vol. 26, 2; pp 223–30.

Young, M. W. *The Ethnography of Malinowski: The Trobriand Islands 1915–18*. Routledge and Kegan Paul, 1979.

Zax, M., Sameroff, A. J. & Farnum, J. E. 'Childbirth education, maternal attitudes and delivery.' *American Journal of Obstetrics and Gynecology*, September 1975; pp 185–90.

Zimmerman-Tansella *et al*. 'Preparation courses for childbirth in primipara: a comparison.' *Journal of Psychosomatic Research*, Vol. 23; pp 227–33.

THE BIRTH TRADITIONS
SURVIVAL BANK

•

As a result of her research in south east Asia and writing this book Jacky Vincent Priya decided to set up the Birth Traditions Survival Bank which is a multifaceted collection of information from all over the world about the traditions associated with conception, pregnancy, birth and the neonatal period. It consists of:

- A computerized data base of articles and books about birth traditions worldwide.

- A photographic picture library together with artistic, literary and other works of relevant interest.

- Empirical data from research carried out specifically for the Bank and from women who have experienced various birth traditions either individually or professionally.

The aims of the Birth Traditions Survival Bank are:

- To bring together a wealth of diverse and scattered information about birth traditions worldwide.

- To carry out empirical research on birth traditions before they are forgotten and lost forever.

- To make this data accessible to everyone from pregnant women wanting to know about their own traditions to the health care professional or politician wanting to integrate traditional practitioners into a woman centred health service for women and children.

Anyone interested in the British Traditions Survival Bank can become part of the Network and receive a quarterly Newsletter. It cost £20/US35 per year to subscribe and further details can be obtained from Jacky Vincent Priya, at the following address.

The Birth Traditions Survival Bank
Private Bag 2
Mtunthama
Malawi
Central Africa

The Bank is always interested in hearing from anyone who, through experience or through their professional work, has come in contact with birth traditions old and new. If you have any information like this or if you are carrying out research on this or any allied topic do please write.

INDEX